Sexual
Intelligence

Sexual Intelligence

What We Really Want from Sex—
and How to Get It

Marty Klein, Ph.D.

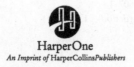

HarperOne
An Imprint of HarperCollinsPublishers

HarperOne

SEXUAL INTELLIGENCE: *What We Really Want from Sex—and How to Get It.*

HarperCollins books may be purchased for educational, business, or sales promotional use. For information, please e-mail the Special Markets Department at SPsales@harpercollins.com.

HarperCollins website: http://www.harpercollins.com

HarperCollins®, 🦅®, and HarperOne™ are trademarks of HarperCollins Publishers.

FIRST HARPERCOLLINS PAPERBACK EDITION PUBLISHED IN 2012

Library of Congress Cataloging-in-Publication Data
 Klein, Marty.
 Sexual intelligence : what we really want from sex—and how to get it /
 by Marty Klein. — 1st ed.
     p.   cm.
   ISBN 978–0–06–202607–1
   1. Sex.   2. Sex instruction.   I. Title.
 HQ21.K5344   2012
 613.9'6—dc23   2011019099

HB 12.06.2022

Contents

Part Three
Implications and Applications

Acknowledgments

Endless conversations and thinking about sex: this may sound like the ideal life, and maybe it is. But it's also very hard work. Understanding one of the most bedeviling and beguiling topics in all of human experience is difficult enough. Attempting to shape that understanding into recognizable ideas, and to communicate those ideas in compelling, new, and helpful ways—now that is frustrating, often overwhelming, very hard work. It may be the ideal life, but don't romanticize the work.

Fortunately, I don't have to do it alone. I have generous partners for those endless conversations, smart and experienced professionals who eagerly consider my latest thoughts. This book is informed by dozens and dozens and dozens of late-night, early-morning, and creative "what if" conversations. And so I thank my partners-in-thought: Vena Blanchard, Doug Braun-Henry, Larry Hedges, Dagmar Herzog, Paul Joannides, and Charles Moser.

And while we don't talk often enough, I always learn something when I discuss the intersections of culture and sexuality with my pals Ellyn Bader, Mickey Diamond, Bill Fisher, Melissa Fritchle, Meg Kaplan, Dick Krueger, Janet Lever, Deb Levine, Peter Pearson, Pepper Schwartz, Bill Taverner, and Carol Tavris. Megan Andelloux made helpful comments on an early draft.

Susan Boyd has generously helped me understand the relevance of my work in the new world of social media. Looking at my work through her insightful, worldly eyes has taught me a great deal.

Veronica Randall has once again shaped my thinking, and therefore my writing. In the early stages of this book, she succeeded in showing me what wouldn't work. As always, she did it as gently as you'd handle a squirmy lamb.

Michael Castleman is a special friend and colleague (and a great writer). I know he doesn't exactly mean to, but he's constantly demanding that I clarify what I want, what I'm trying to say, and why. The constancy of his affection and respect regardless of my answers makes his questions all the more powerful. He's also done more to ease me into the post-print world of writing than anyone else.

Doug Kirby and Jack Morin are highly accomplished and dear friends. Their confidence in my ability has helped me through more than one bout of wondering what, exactly, was the point of writing yet another book. For decades we have been investigating both sexuality and life together. As a result, I am a better sexologist and a better man.

Eric Brandt brought the book to HarperOne. During his tenure with me, his hand was warm and valuable.

I very much appreciate my editor, Cindy DiTiberio. With enthusiasm and insight, she did something that all editors attempt and few accomplish—she made this book better.

If I wore a hat, I'd gratefully tip it to my agent, Will Lippincott. Will is an old-fashioned gentleman, with a thoroughly modern sensibility. On my behalf, he elegantly navigates the world's most arcane industry with an uncanny understanding of both it and me. We are a distinctly odd couple—and he generously, graciously, makes it work for both of us.

And my wife? My patient, insightful, literate, loving wife? Aw, don't get me started; that would take a whole other book. All I'll say is, if you knew her, you'd envy me.

Sexual Intelligence

Introduction

No Wonder Most People Don't

True or False?

(Answers appear on page 7.)

- You can now buy vibrators, handcuffs, dildos, and anal beads on Amazon.com.

- Eighty-six percent of American adults say they masturbate.

- Although millions of men get a prescription for Viagra, Cialis, or Levitra every year, the number of men who renew their prescription is very low.

- People into S/M—spanking, whipping, blindfolding, etc.—are no more likely to come from abusive backgrounds than non-S/Mers.

- Many men of all ages don't ejaculate every time they have sex—and many women consider themselves a failure when this happens.

- In 2010, only 20 percent of a university student sample said that oral sex is "sex."

- More money was spent on pornography in the United States last year than on tickets for all professional baseball, football, basketball, and hockey games combined.

- More than one million Americans went to a swingers' club last year.

- Half of all mass market paperbacks sold in the United States are romance novels. Last year half of all American adults read at least one romance novel. The average reader of romance novels reads *fifty* per year.

- Most school sex education programs in the United States are not allowed to use the words *clitoris* or *pleasure*.

Sex isn't just an activity—it's an idea.

Our ideas about sex are so complicated that we make the activity complicated. I'm here to make both your ideas and your sexual activity *less* complicated. In my thirty-plus years as a sex therapist and marriage counselor, this almost always makes sex easier and more enjoyable. In many cases, more frequent, too.

When we're young, sexual desire is driven by hormones, lust, hunger, novelty, and an urge to prove ourselves. Most of us are soooooo horny. We desire the most profound—and primitive—fusion with our lust object. If only we could unzip our torso and he or she could climb right in!

We're told that eventually, desire will be driven, not by hormones, but by love. We plan to feel, one day, "You're so great, so perfect for me, I want you."

And eventually most of us do fall in love. We idealize our partner. And typically, we're horny for him or her.

As the relationship continues to evolve, both partners finally get to know each other. Routine sets in. If we want novelty, we must create it—a weekend in the country, new furniture, new fantasies. And we stop idealizing our partner. Once we do, love no longer triggers desire reliably, because the rest of life interferes.

Sex becomes less frequent. Or more routine. Or both.

When a relationship is new and the sex is exotic and enjoyable, the start-up cost of each sexual encounter is low. We're not nervous about hearing "no," and we're usually not nervous about hearing "yes." But as sex becomes less frequent, we feel increasingly awkward. Starting up each sexual encounter becomes more complex, more time-consuming, more fraught with anxiety.

The hassle of initiating sex starts to outweigh the perceived advantages of having it. If a couple gets along, they have other, dependable ways to enjoy themselves: a walk, cooking together, watching TV, napping, photographing their kids, playing Scrabble. When a couple has limited free time together and they know they can reliably have fun doing other things, choosing to have sex that they imagine might involve self-consciousness, disappointment, criticism, and emotional distance is simply irrational.

So long-term couples who like each other do the most obvious thing: they have sex less often, and instead do other things they enjoy more easily.

If you and your partner want sex to be part of your lives after the first few years, you can't rely on feeling hormonal lust, you can't rely on feeling overwhelmed by being in love, and you can't rely on feeling there's nothing better to do. The two of you have to do something fundamentally irrational—propose something that's less enjoyable and more emotionally expensive than practically any other leisure activity available.

And what about the actual sex you are going to have when you get around to having it?

Every one of us learns about sex when we have the body of a young person. By the time we're thirty, virtually no one has that body anymore. And forty? You can look fantastic. You can have great style, that special something that still attracts attention. But you no longer have the body you had when you were learning about sex. The body you have now behaves differently, doesn't it?

If you use your young adult vision of sex with your mature body, you're going to have trouble. And your emotions will rebel: if sex means, for example, instant wetness, rock-hard erection, pounding intercourse, and simultaneous orgasm, you will feel anxious about failing—and that's another reason to not initiate sex, or to not respond when your partner does.

On the other hand, if you put together a different vision of sex that is attuned to your current situation—a body with a few dings, a partner who isn't young, limitations of time and place, emotional scars—you'll be more willing to initiate, since your chance of a satisfying encounter is much greater. That means you have to change a few of your ideas about the meaning of desire and arousal, of sexual "function" and "dysfunction."

In fact, you have to change the way you think about sex.

Of course, changing your vision of sex can feel uncomfortable—"If I were still young I wouldn't have to change my vision," or, "If I were still great in bed I wouldn't have to change my vision"—and so you have to come to terms with this necessity. If you do, *and* you change your vision, *and* you're willing to push yourself to participate, *and* your expectations are different, *and* you have a sense of humor and some humility, you might create something enjoyable.

No wonder so many people don't.

———

In this book, you'll meet more than three dozen of my patients. They're nice people (well, mostly), but they make sex difficult for themselves. They make it about being normal, about hiding, about romance, about being young, about perfection, about being womanly, about desperately trying not to fail.

So of course they feel intimidated, resentful, pessimistic, enervated. And they blame: they blame sex, women, pornography, menopause, the economy, their small breasts, "stress." I like most of my patients, but I'm afraid it's people like these who give sex a bad name.

My patients want sex to be "natural" and "spontaneous," to "just happen." Many reject the idea of putting effort into creating adult sex, so they just retreat into adolescent sex—affairs, romance novels, Internet chat, constant pornography, low desire.

But it's time for us all to grow up and relearn how to experience our sexuality. It's time for Sexual Intelligence. What is that?

Sexual Intelligence =
Information + Emotional Skills + Body Awareness

Here's a preview of this idea:

- Sexual Intelligence is the ability to keep sex in perspective regardless of what happens during sex.

- To get more out of sex, we have to change. To change we need a different perspective. Sexual Intelligence is that perspective.

- Sexual Intelligence is useful in different ways at different times of life: in our twenties, in exploring the sexual world; in our thirties, in bonding with a partner and establishing a sexual rhythm; in our forties, in tolerating and adapting to change; in our fifties, in saying good-bye to youthful sex; in our sixties and beyond, in creating a new sexual style.

This is good news—it helps explain why you may not have been able to improve sex (because you haven't been changing your paradigm), and it should give you hope that there's something you haven't tried that might work.

The Sexual Intelligence perspective predicts and explains some of the key features of contemporary sexuality:

- Why Viagra doesn't help a lot of people, even though it gives them erections

- Why learning new positions doesn't improve frustrating sex

- Why desire problems are the most common issue people bring to sex therapy

- Why desire problems are sex therapy's unresolved treatment challenge

- Why Internet porn use has risen astronomically, and why so many people make or enjoy amateur porn

- Why most people feel so bad when they're sexually dissatisfied

Sexual Intelligence allows us to use sexuality to express ourselves authentically. We can have sex without it, of course, but it won't necessarily reflect who we are (or think we are). When we are sexually dissatisfied, we typically don't look at our Sexual Intelligence. We try to fix the wrong things—erections, orgasms, lubrication, an aging body—but even if these fixes are successful, that usually doesn't make the sex more enjoyable. It's like trying to teach a pig to sing: you ultimately don't accomplish what you want, and it mostly just annoys the pig.

Sexual Intelligence is what gets you from adolescent sex to adult sex. It's what gets you from hormone-driven sex to sex you choose. It's what gets you from "sex has to validate me" to "I validate my sexuality." It's what allows you to adapt sex to yourself, instead of you adapting to sex.

After thirty years of listening to sexually frustrated, unhappy, confused, resentful, anxious, impulsive, and self-critical people, I've noticed the similarities in all that unsatisfying sex. But satisfying, life-affirming sex is different. It comes in an infinite number of flavors, created anew by each person and each couple. Let's find out what *your* version is—and how to use your Sexual Intelligence to create it.

Answers to quiz on page 1:
Each of these ten statements is true.

Part One

Telling the Truth About Sex

Chapter One

What Do People Say
They Want from Sex?
What Do They *Really* Want?

Carlton came to see me with a simple question: "Why don't I want to have intercourse?"

Yes, just another day in the office.

Carlton is a retired engineer, a friendly-looking sixty-eight-year-old guy with a quick smile. He told me he had a new girlfriend, Lina—"although 'girlfriend' is a funny word for a sixty-three-year-old woman," he laughed.

Carlton was a year out of a thirty-year-long marriage, which sounded terrible. His wife, Genevieve, disappointed that her career in real estate never took off and that she never had kids, had turned bitter and cold decades before. He had withdrawn—first from her, then from life in general. Week after week, he spent his time working and avoiding Genevieve. Sex had never been central to their marriage, and they soon stopped.

When Genevieve finally divorced him in disgust, he was left alone. About eight months later, he met Lina through a friend. "I couldn't believe it," he beamed. "She was warm, friendly, colorful, so full of life." They had lunch a few times, and eventually were spending every afternoon together. Then it was every evening, too.

"She loved to kiss, she said I was good at it," he said shyly, not quite looking at me. No one had said that to him since he was eighteen. "So soon we were doing other physical things, and eventually we were sexual in lots of different ways. We'd spend all morning fooling around. It was great!"

In the afternoons they'd go out into the world—hiking, biking, seeing old movies, going to museums. He rediscovered his love of music. It was a delirious time. She helped him buy some new, more stylish clothes. "Look, I'm wearing a silk shirt," he smiled. "And she dresses up for me, even around the house. Fabulous!"

But she wanted intercourse. He didn't. She asked why. He didn't know. She suggested he see me.

"So why don't I want intercourse?" he asked.

"Why do you think you don't want intercourse?" I responded.

"Well, Lina's counselor says I'm probably afraid of intimacy. And I saw a therapist for a few sessions before seeing you—she says I'm hesitant to assume my manly role in this relationship, especially after being emasculated in my marriage."

"Is that what you think?"

"Um, it doesn't really sound right, but I don't know. Doesn't everyone want intercourse? Lina's so hot for it. She swears I'll love it. What's wrong with me?"

"Well," I said, turning the conventional wisdom upside down, "why should you want intercourse?"

"I never thought of that. Doesn't everyone?"

"We're not here to discuss everyone, Carlton, just you. You're not trying to conceive, are you?" We both chuckled. "Then why should intercourse be special, why should it be at the top of some hierarchy?"

"This is pretty strange talk," he announced, but he was intrigued.

"You're having the best sex of your life, right, Carlton?"

"Right."

"You're having a great time, almost every day you're kissing and touching a lovely nude woman who's energetic and enthusiastic, right?"

"Right."

"You're both having orgasms and pleasure, and you're looking at each other the whole time. Why change anything?"

He thought about it for a while. Then he said quietly, "She's the one who wants me to want intercourse. She says she wants to feel desired, and that's how a woman knows a man desires her. But of course I desire her! I tell her constantly, and we're always having sex, even if I'm not totally in the mood."

Carlton was no "lazy lover," and he loved sex and intimacy with Lina. But as he started paying more attention to his actual experience with her, he realized he was feeling bossed around. "And she's nervous about why I don't want to screw," he said. "I'm getting tired of reassuring her."

Lina kept saying she wanted Carlton to make love to her "like a man." "I don't really go for that," he frowned. It seemed clear to me he wasn't *afraid* of being "manly"—he just didn't find it very entertaining. As her sense of urgency about this increased, he found himself increasingly resentful—and that scared him.

"Carlton, you're like Sleeping Beauty," I said. "Your months with Lina have woken you up, which is glorious. At first you welcomed her as your guide back into life. Now you're becoming more independent, and some of Lina's rigidities and insecurities are losing their charm."

"Yes," he nodded vigorously. "It's my life, and I don't have to do everything her way—in fact, I want to keep some of my old shirts!" We both laughed.

"I'm nervous about confronting her," he continued. "I want to be with her, but I can't let her tell me how to make love. And I can't let her bully me into being her kind of man."

In fact, they almost broke up when Carlton started setting some limits with Lina. But after weeks of quarreling, they understood themselves and each other a lot better.

"When intercourse isn't loaded down with all this pressure and meaning, I might find it more interesting," he said. "For now, we've agreed that great sex is more important than what kind of great sex. At least, she says we can do that for a while, and then we can talk again."

✳ ✳ ✳

What People Say

What do most men and women say they want from sex?

On the one hand, various people mention a broad range of things: orgasm, "intimacy," feeling desired, a great blow job, lots of kissing, a hard penis, light spanking, and satisfying their partner, to name a few.

On the other hand, almost everyone's answer comes down to this: *what most people say they want from sex is some combination of pleasure and closeness.*

Yet, as a sex therapist, I can tell you that that's *not* what most people focus on during sex. Think about it—do you?

So what do people—what do you—focus on during sex instead?

- How they look
- How they smell
- How they sound
- Preventing unwanted activity (for example, having their shoulder bitten)
- Ignoring (or preventing) pain
- Hurrying to climax
- Trying not to climax too quickly
- Maintaining an erection or lubrication
- Suppressing emotions
- Trying to function "the right way"
- Silently, indirectly urging their partner to do a certain activity (such as stroking their clitoris)

It's not surprising that if people say they want one thing from sex and then spend the experience focused on everything *except* that, they'll be dissatisfied.

But people say they focus on those other things (like how they look, or suppressing their emotions) *in order* to have better sex. "I don't want him turned off by my big butt," some women say, "so I usually don't let him get me from behind." I've heard men say things like, "I'm always afraid she feels bored while she's giving me oral sex, so I guess I'm constantly checking—is she frowning, does she seem uncomfortable?"

In the quest for sexual satisfaction, many people especially insist on focusing on how their genitalia are working: "I need to know

I'm gonna stay hard long enough for my wife to be satisfied," or, "When I think I'm taking too long to climax, I hurry up, or even fake it."

Most people don't think of this as a distraction, but it is—bigger than dirty dishes or unpaid bills could ever be. *Focusing on how your penis or vulva is working is an enormous distraction from pursuing pleasure or intimacy.* Although many people think that's the way to make sex better, I'm afraid they're exactly wrong.

A lot of people (and a lot of therapists) apparently don't understand that. When people come to my office, they never say, "Please help me stop focusing on my erections, my orgasms, my desire to function the right way—it's preventing me from enjoying sex." No, if anything, they want me to help them do those things *better*. "Doc, how can I make us climax at the same time?" "Doc, how do I stay hard during oral sex even when she's being too rough?"

Helping people identify what they're actually thinking about during sex is powerful. Helping them realize that their thoughts are often obstacles to satisfaction is even more powerful.

Many people are *watching* themselves during sex more than they are *experiencing* sex, which typically undermines sexual enjoyment. We usually imagine, harshly judge, and worry about what our partner sees, smells, hears, and tastes. This is far more distracting than thinking about work or laundry. Because once sex becomes about how we appear to others, we can't stop monitoring ourselves. We're constantly making decisions about how authentic to be, and how much to pose. (This is one reason men and women fake orgasms.) This continual vigilance dramatically disrupts our erotic feelings, expression, and satisfaction.

It's like trying to enjoy dinner while wearing a brand-new expensive white suit. Even if you succeed in keeping the suit clean, constantly paying attention to it eventually takes over, and ruins, the meal.

Okay, so we focus on other stuff. Why?

Whether it's our big bellies or our increasingly gray pubic hair or our no-longer-quite-so-perky breasts (remember, breasts don't *sag* as we get older, they *relax*), whether it's our concern about keeping an erection long after our partner has had enough thrusting, or our fear of smelling bad while our partner goes down on us, why do we focus on extraneous stuff like this during sex?

One reason is that we think this is where sexiness lives or dies, and we think "sexiness" is crucial to satisfaction. We'll address this damaging (and incorrect) belief soon enough. But another reason is that there are, after all, other things we want from sex besides pleasure and closeness.

For most women and men, those needs can include:

- Reassurance that we're sexually desirable

- Reassurance that we're sexually competent

- Validation of our masculinity or femininity

- A sense that we're normal

- Relief from performance anxiety

. . . and so on.

A lot of our behavior around sex is designed to address these other needs, whether we acknowledge them or not. As we'll see, our strategies usually aren't successful, but we use them anyway. And it turns out that we're putting a lot of pressure on sex to address these essentially non-sexual needs. To put it another way, most of us have emotional needs that we try to address with sex, but sex is *not* the best way to satisfy them.

For some people, reassurance, validation, and relief are the real payoffs of sex. Sure, pleasure and closeness are great, but they can't compete with feeling whole, feeling real, feeling normal, and feeling "I'm good enough and I can relax for a minute." And I've learned that that's what many people are trying to accomplish via sex.

I'm not saying that people *don't* want pleasure or closeness from sex. Most people do want some combination of pleasure and closeness from sex—*after* their other emotional needs are met.

People don't necessarily know this about themselves. But if you're struggling with these emotional needs, pursuing them through performance-oriented sex, and you don't realize it, you may feel that sex is more trouble than it's worth, or that feeling alone during sex is normal, or that sex is not the time to feel like yourself.

That's what my patients usually mean when they say things like, "Sex isn't as great as it used to be," or, "Something's missing from sex, and I'm not sure what it is."

Attempting to indirectly get validation, reassurance, and other psychological fulfillment from sex—especially if we don't admit our agenda to ourselves or inform our partner—makes sex complicated, unpredictable, and a lot of work. We make it even harder on ourselves by creating narrow, rigid definitions of the satisfactions we seek; if "manliness" means always being erect regardless of fatigue, for instance, or "competent" means climaxing every time, sexual "success" will be frustratingly elusive.

Perhaps this helps explain why you aren't focused on pleasure and closeness during sex. It's because you're also looking for something else, whether you know it or not. This also helps explain why so many people are sexually dissatisfied—because sex isn't delivering what they really want, in fact *can't* deliver what they want through genital excellence. And any psychological satisfaction you accidentally get doesn't stick to your ribs because it's indirect, unacknowledged, and fleeting.

If you don't tell your partner about this other agenda, it's easy to feel alone during sex. And of course, it's harder to create the sex you want when you don't involve your partner directly.

If you're someone who wants more "communication" around sex, this is a good place to start: tell your partner that you want more from sex than just amazing orgasms (whether you currently have them or not). But make it clear that you're not asking your partner to "give" you a good emotional experience (that does sound like drudgery); tell your partner that you see your sex life as a collaboration, and that you realize you need to step up a bit too.

My patient Craig, for example, felt intimidated by his new girlfriend's very active sexual past. Although Ellie was open with him about it, he always felt there was more to her story. It didn't help that he hadn't gotten over his first wife's infidelity before he became involved with someone new.

What Craig really wanted to hear was that he was the best lover Ellie ever had—partly because he felt competitive with all her previous partners, and partly because he feared losing her the way he'd lost his first wife.

But he never told Ellie this in a simple, straightforward way. After they would make love (three or four times most weeks), he'd always ask if she enjoyed it, if she climaxed (as if he couldn't see or hear it himself!), if she was satisfied. Not that she was shy about her enjoyment, but getting her to say yes, yes, yes, was his way of arranging to feel sexually competent and important. Although he didn't admit it to himself until our therapy, this was just as important to him as the intimacy or pleasure he felt from making love with Ellie.

Performance Anxiety

For many people, sex is mostly about success and failure: whether or not they unintentionally hurt, disappoint, or annoy their partner; or expose themselves as inadequate or inexperienced; or make a fool of themselves. Frequently people are concerned that their body won't do what it "should" (like get an erection) or that it will do what it "shouldn't" (like wet the bed). For millions of men and women, "I didn't mess that up too badly" is as good as sex gets.

As we'll see later, one of the wonderful things about sex is that we can make it a place where mistakes are simply not possible, and where virtually nothing can go wrong—not because we become sexually perfect, but because we radically redefine sexual "success."

Meanwhile, here are the sounds of "performance anxiety," straight from my patients. Perhaps you've said or thought one or more of these yourself, anxious that you might not "perform" as expected by either your partner or yourself:

- "She's expecting sex on her birthday—and I can't guarantee I'll be in the mood."

- "I can't compete with Megan Fox or Angelina Jolie."

- "We went out last week with a couple that just fell in love. It's intimidating to be with people so hot for each other."

- "Oprah says if you can't get it up, it's either my fault or your fault."

- "My girlfriend just lost weight and bought lingerie—what if I'm not interested enough?"

- "It's been a perfect Saturday night—I'd hate to ruin it by agreeing to have sex and then coming too soon."

- "He hasn't had sex in a week, and tomorrow the kids return from camp."

- "That film we saw last week turned out to be really sexy, and we were both squirming uncomfortably."

Most people want to "perform" well during sex, imagining that it's the best way to create satisfaction (and avoid "failure" and their partner's disappointment). But especially since so much of sexual "performance" is beyond our control (we can't will an erection or lubrication), the need to "perform" well leads to anxiety. Ironically, feeling pressure to perform "successfully" during sex creates and maintains much of the sexual difficulty and frustration that people fear, and ultimately have. People crave relief from this pressure, while lamenting that relief is impossible.

Of course, pursuing relief from performance anxiety by attempting to perform better is exactly the wrong way to do it—but clearly that's what many people imagine will work. We can laugh at the superstitions of star athletes: Michael Jordan wearing his North Carolina shorts under his Bulls uniform every game, or Peyton Manning reading the stadium program cover to cover before every game. But while these rituals are harmless, focusing on sexual performance isn't—in fact, it often makes our "performance" worse. Imagine how quickly Michael Jordan would ditch those shorts if he knew they were undermining his shooting!

Today's self-help industry, psychology and medical experts, and marriage revival workshops—not to mention Victoria's Secret—ignore this basic truth. They try to help people have better sex by leaving their faulty assumptions and rigid definitions in place, simply adding gender myths and sunny "you can do it" encouragement on top of them. But like constructing a building on a shaky foundation, it's a mistake, one that makes the sexual "failure" people fear almost inevitable. That's why so much of my caseload is people who have "failed" with other therapists and programs.

And then "women" are blamed. Or "men" are blamed. Or sex is blamed. While we're at it, let's remember to blame pornography, stress, menopause, "you've gained weight," and all that email that's always piling up.

Attempting to resolve emotional issues around sex by trying to have amazing sex is like attempting to resolve the emotional needs we bring to athletics by trying to be an amazing athlete.

When my patient Juan was a kid, he was terrible at sports. He wanted to please his father, a soccer player who treated his physically awkward son harshly. In response, of course, Juan always tried too hard, which made playing well even more difficult—and even if he had played well, there's no way he could have enjoyed it. As a child, Juan had emotional needs connected with sports—feeling worthy of his father's love, feeling connected with others his age—that he couldn't satisfy.

Rather than using sports as the way to address these internal issues, Juan might have used a different vehicle (interesting conversation, a shared hobby, pride in a career)—*except that he was a kid*. Understandably, he believed that both his pain and its solution were located in sports.

As an adult, Juan should now realize that weekend athletics are just for fun, but they still feel terribly important to him, and it drives him crazy when he doesn't succeed. That's because the emotional pairing he learned in childhood is embedded in Juan's unconscious.

Would you have told young Juan that the answer to his problems with his father was to be a better athlete? Of course not. What about the adult Juan—would you tell him to just work harder and become a better athlete, or would you suggest something more psychologically sophisticated?

That's the position many people are in about sexuality. They're trying to resolve one or another psychological problem by trying to create amazing sex. And it simply doesn't work. I know most people think the way to resolve the emotional needs they bring to sex is by having amazing sex. Unfortunately, most media shrinks and clinical professionals agree.

They're wrong.

Besides, you can't even have amazing sex when you're focused on other emotional needs (especially if they're unconscious). That's like expecting to enjoy a concert or play when you're afraid everyone's staring at you, smirking at what you're wearing. And so people pursue amazing sex, but they get neither their emotional *nor* their sexual needs met. And then they're really disappointed—and often angry or self-critical as well.

So let's go back to what people really want from sex.

Most people don't talk about this accurately—either because they don't have the vocabulary or because they're embarrassed, hesitant, or scared to use words. (What's *your* reason?) If people did talk about what they want from sex thoroughly and accurately, they'd use language that's primarily experiential rather than functional. That is, instead of talking about what their bodies might *do*, they'd talk about how they would like to *feel*.

And how do people want to feel before, during, after, and with regard to sex? My clinical experience suggests that people want to feel . . .

- Un-self-conscious

- Youthful

- Graceful

- Passionate

- Like they have all the time in the world

- Attractive

- Competent

- Special

- Like they're inventing sex

- Unintimidated

All this does sound great, doesn't it? The challenge is to create such experiences *while you relax*. Otherwise, there's a limit to how much you can enjoy such feelings. After all, how much can you enjoy being told you're attractive when you're afraid you'll wet the bed or lose your erection?

Changing Your Sexual Vision

Put another way, during sex people want to feel the way they felt when they were emerging adults. Or the way they imagine other young adults felt. And so they say things about sex like:

- "I want spontaneity."
- "I don't want to communicate—I just want to do it and have everything work fine."
- "Why can't sex just be natural? I hate the way it's all complicated now."
- "Thinking too much about sex takes away the romance, the mystery."
- "Talking too much about sex makes it mechanical."

Listening to feelings like these, anyone would think that eroticism is so delicate and ephemeral that it disappears if we shine any light on it, or mention it above a whisper. And yet I understand people's anxiety, frustration, and resentment about this. For many men and women, sex seemed so easy when they were younger, and it seems so much more complicated now.

Early adulthood (roughly age eighteen to twenty-five) is the time when most people are settling into their sexual identities, typically wrestling with questions like: Who am I regarding sex? What's my relationship to sexuality? What will its role in my life be? What do sexual satisfaction and sexual frustration feel like? What are reasonable responses to each?

It's while you have a young body and youthful lifestyle that you're making your most serious decisions about sex: What does "horny" feel like? How do men really feel about women who love sex? Is birth control really important? What kind of sex is manly? Is oral sex really sex? Answer a few hundred questions like these—remember, with the perspective of a youthful body and lifestyle—and that's your sexual identity, your vision of what it means for you to be sexual.

Logically, as both our bodies and lifestyles change, our sexual vision needs to change too. After all, most of us tend to change our vision and self-image about other important things, such as work, food, family, and health. But many people, misled by the media, the fashion industry, "successful aging" psychologists, and others, don't change their sexual vision over time—and that means trouble.

A lot of my patients have difficulty reconciling a sexual vision that's ten or twenty or thirty years out of date with a body and lifestyle that can't support that vision comfortably. Rather than challenge and reshape the vision, most of them say that there's something wrong with themselves or their partner, and they want me to fix one or both.

There's no lack of therapists (or TV commercials for drugs, cosmetics, and alcohol) who agree that such people have a "dysfunction." But pursuing a sexual vision that's fifteen years out of date (and performing poorly at it!) isn't a "dysfunction." It's a culturally and psychologically driven mistake.

Instead, I point out to my patients what their sexual vision is—the gender stereotypes, the myths about intercourse or orgasm, the assumption that loneliness during sex is inevitable. I help them see how such a vision is obsolete, and I help them craft a new one. This is where Sexual Intelligence is helpful. We deal with their grief, sadness, anger, or despair about letting go of old sexual dreams—so they can eventually create new, more realistic ones.

People no longer young (that's most adults) often want a sex life that matches the one they had—or wanted to have, or believe they should have had—when they were young. And that's what much of the self-help industry sells—sex like when we were young. (There's even a ridiculous new book called *Have Sex Like You Just Met . . . No Matter How Long You've Been Together,* by two writers with no credentials whatsoever. With a title like that, of course, the book will sell plenty. Can a Jennifer Aniston film be far behind?)

It doesn't work. It can't.

No, sex isn't going to be like it was when you were young—if by "when I was young" you mean endless physical energy, hormone-crazed lust, all the time in the world, self-indulgent impulsivity with no sense of the consequences, and a partner who's young and also wild with hormones. No, sex is not going to be like that regularly ever again.

Unless, of course, you have a continuing series of new partners or take really wild risks that get your adrenaline pumping. But that isn't how most adults want to live—do you?

Sorry to deliver the news so directly. Psychologist Irvin Yalom, who unblinkingly challenges patients to see themselves and their relationships clearly, was once called "Love's Executioner" (now the title of his 1989 classic book). Sometimes my patients call me similar names. Like "Youth's Executioner." Or the "Grim Speaker." They're mostly grateful to hear the truth, but they hate hearing it just the same.

All of this being said, sex can be deeply satisfying—pleasurable, fun, intimate—if you want. But you may have to change your ideas about satisfaction. You need to either want different things, or to redefine the things you continue to want.

You can, for example, feel graceful, youthful, competent, timeless, and un-self-conscious during sex. All you have to do is make room in this definition for imperfect bodies and imperfect "function" (unlike when you were younger). If your back hurts, you go slow instead of pounding your partner and hurting yourself. If you tend to wet the bed, you put a towel down instead of distracting yourself by thinking about wetting the bed. If you like lots of kissing, you ask for (and you do) lots of kissing, rather than wishing for it. If a spanking is more exciting than kissing, you ask for that instead.

If you're taking a medication that makes your mouth dry, you put a glass of water on the night table and you use it during sex. Ditto lube. If your breasts have, um, relaxed over time, you deal with it—once and for all, because they're not going to magically get perky overnight. Finish dealing with that issue now, and your breasts will never be an obstacle to enjoying sex ever again.

We'll discuss how to implement a new sexual vision in Part Three.

So that's it: Sexual Intelligence means dealing with sexuality in a straightforward way, rather than hiding it, denying it, or blaming it. You talk about it. You don't put your energy into pretending that sex isn't the way it is.

A few years ago, I taught a sexuality seminar for student therapists at a fancy southern university. When they couldn't quite understand this idea, I used the analogy of having people over to your home for dinner. I said that, when inviting someone, a good host asks, "Is there anything you don't eat?" A good guest tells the truth, responding that he or she is allergic to shellfish or almonds or whatever. Then the host can cook something the guest will like, and neither guest nor cook will be disappointed or embarrassed.

One of the students scoffed at my vision. "If I invite you to dinner, I don't ask any questions," she said. "I make what I want, and you eat it or not!" Well, I don't want to unfairly generalize as to sex—but I certainly wouldn't want to go to that young woman's house for dinner—would you?

A Means, Not an End

Like most people, you probably assume that creating enjoyable sex requires that your penis or vulva do the various tricks it did (or was supposed to do) when you were younger. But remember, *sexual function is a means to an end, not an end in itself.* People talk about erections, lubrication, and orgasm as if those are the point of sex. But this vision of sex is way too limited.

Of course, if one of your primary goals in sex is to "not mess up too badly," I understand why you have this focus. If you believe that getting your body to do what it used to do (or never did, but "should" do) is what constitutes "successful" sex, of course you'll get attached to those particular abilities. But unlike many therapists, I don't support people's attachment to the functioning they believe creates sexual success—I treat that attachment *as a problem*.

So a key part of Sexual Intelligence is realizing that your body is not going to have sex like it did when you were younger. Some people find this unacceptable; they'd rather be unhappy and still hold out the hope of regaining (or creating) their sexual youth instead of changing internally and learning how to enjoy sex. After all, most people would rather have and keep a temporary problem than have and accept a permanent problem.

For some people, rejecting this insight is part of their larger (usually unconscious) project of denying their aging or impending death. This can go on with thirty-year-olds as much as with sixty-year-olds. People with this project have bigger fish to fry than sex. They're dealing with the most serious existential issue there is.

I'm very sympathetic about people's desire for passion. As we'll see throughout this book, passion is possible—but it will probably look different than you thought it would. When adults experience passion, it's usually not in response to incredible sex or the perfect body—it's usually in response to giving themselves permission to let go emotionally. More on that as we go along.

There's one more concern people have about being sexually relaxed and authentic. It's terribly distracting, and it inhibits people before, during, and after sex. You might recognize it in yourself—the desire to be sexually normal, and the suspicion (or outright anxiety) that you're not. In the next chapter, we'll look at normality anxiety in detail.

Chapter Two

Am I Normal?

*Why Focusing on "Normal Sex"
Undermines Sex*

Forty-year-olds Thomas and Danni—a high school
teacher and accountant, respectively—had many of
the things most couples want. But not sex.

And that's why they came to me. "We love each other, but
no one ever initiates sex," he said. "Yes," she added, "and
when we have sex, it's tense, we're nervous, it's over pretty
quick. It isn't fun like it should be."

Well, that explains why no one initiates, I thought. Love
won't get people into bed too often if the sex mostly just
gets on their nerves.

Thomas and Danni clearly enjoyed the small amount of
time they had together (she worked Saturdays and two
evenings each week, while his hours were the usual Monday
through Friday), but the lack of sex hung over their lives like
a damp gray haze. I asked each of them why they didn't initiate, and their answers were similar: "We're uptight," Danni

said. "We're stressed," Thomas said. "We're just not in the habit of it," Danni said. "We're so busy, and by the time bedtime comes, we're just too tired," Thomas said.

"Notice all the 'we' and the lack of 'I'?" I asked. "Let's try it again. I'd like you each to tell me why *you* don't initiate sex." After a nervous silence, they did. "I'm afraid I won't get a good enough erection," Thomas said shyly. "And if I do, that I'll come too fast and Danni will be disappointed. And I'm concerned that if I make too much noise or get carried away, it will scare her."

Now we were getting somewhere. "Danni?"

"I know he's worried about that stuff," she said. "It makes me sad to see him so worried, so I don't encourage us to make love. Plus, when we do have sex and I see how hard he's trying to please me, I feel guilty."

"So if Thomas weren't concerned about all that, would you be more likely to initiate sex?" I've learned to ask about people's willingness to *initiate* sex, rather than their willingness to *have* sex—I get much more information that way. "Well, even without that. . . ." She too was shy. "See, I don't always orgasm, and I'm afraid he'll be disappointed, so that's usually on my mind when I think about sex. So if I'm tired or there's some other reason I don't think I'll come, or that it will take a long time, I don't initiate." And then she blurted out, "He really deserves a better sex partner than me!"

There was plenty to work with here. I was glad for them that their health insurance was covering our sessions. It looked like they would need a lot of them.

Thomas and Danni reminded me of the couple in O. Henry's story "The Gift of the Magi." You'll recall that it features a very loving but very poor young couple who want to buy each other a Christmas gift. She cuts off and sells her exquisite hair so she can buy him a chain for his cherished pocket watch; he sells his treasured watch so he can buy her precious combs for her signature hair. Of course, each of them has rendered the other's gift useless, but their love is affirmed.

Well, Thomas and Danni were keeping away from sex because they didn't want to disappoint each other. And they were afraid of disappointing each other because they assumed that sex had to be "normal." If instead of aspiring to normal sex they aspired to sex that was intimate and felt good, they could more easily imagine enjoyable sex together, and maybe even have it on a regular basis, their schedules notwithstanding.

And that's pretty much what I told them.

"If you're trying to create perfect sex, that's going to be intimidating, whether you succeed or fail," I said. "So you need a different goal. Rather than try to create a certain kind of sex, why don't you just make love the way you do other things?" I continued: "How would you characterize the way you do other things together—you know, house projects, going out to dinner, watching DVDs?"

They easily generated and agreed on a half-dozen words: cooperative, fun, respectful, friendly, capable, relaxed. "And sometimes lazy," Thomas added, and they both laughed.

"Great," I said. "You know, not every couple is like this. But since you are, why don't you just make love the way you do everything else?" Such a simple idea, yet so powerful.

Of course they had their objections to this. What if they got into bed, were "just themselves," and nothing happened? What if one of them acted in a really selfish way? What if one of them wanted "kinky stuff"? What if one of them was left unsatisfied?

This is the sound of people defending their soon-to-be obsolete paradigm.

"First," I explained, "neither of you is going to reveal yourself as dramatically different than you already know each other to be. You won't go on some selfish sexual binge because neither of you is terribly selfish. And neither of you will reveal yourself as 'wildly kinky,' because neither of you is an extreme sort of person. Although," I said, with a slight smile, "each of you is a creative type, and maybe sex is a place you've been holding back from each other. That can make sex boring, you know." They looked at each other warmly.

"Second," I continued, "of *course* unexpected things will happen in sex if you're just yourselves. Sometimes you won't want to do the same thing, sometimes one of you will be much more energetic or full of desire than the other, and sometimes nothing will happen—you know, you'll both be lazy and hope the other one will volunteer to do most of the work." They laughed knowingly. We've *all* had that experience.

"The fact that being yourself sometimes leads to the unexpected in sex helps keep sex interesting, which is really important in long-term relationships. And it means that sex is periodically challenging, so it can be a vehicle for personal growth. Since you'll be doing it with someone you really trust, it's a safe medium."

They seemed persuaded. And in the coming weeks they did report an increase in lovemaking—and the fact that they were relaxed, and enjoying it more. "It's like making love with a good friend," said Thomas. "Yes," Danni agreed, "it's like going someplace fun and not worrying, instead of sex being a place where worry is built in."

Perfect. Their vision of sex was changing, so they worked much less at it. And since they found each other attractive and likable, I was certain they'd be having more sex. More importantly, they'd be enjoying it more.

∗ ∗ ∗

What Is Sexually "Normal"?

Here's what's "normal": adults have sex primarily when they're tired.

This shapes the quality, content, and frequency of the experience. Most adults save their "prime time" for things that are either more important (raising their kids, working after hours, maintaining their health, handling crises) or more reliably satisfying (watching TV, going out, sharing hobbies, playing around on Facebook).

Not having much energy is one aspect of "normal sex" that most people *don't* want. But many adults seem to believe that most sex will inevitably take place when they're not at their best, without considering the consequences of this kind of sex life—that it may become routine, not involve much time, lose its playfulness, and that using contraception or a lubricant may seem like too much trouble.

If we think of "normal" as common, typical, and accepted as "the way things are," this is what "normal sex" actually looks like:

- Awkwardness and self-consciousness are common.

- Communication is limited.

- Neither partner laughs or smiles much.

- One or both partners are obsessively concerned about performance.

- One or both are unsure what their partner likes.

- One or both tolerate what they dislike, hoping that it will stop soon.

- Masturbation is kept secret.

- There's difficulty using birth control without embarrassment or conflict.

- Desire requires a perfect environment.

- Sex is sometimes physically painful.

- He believes that "her orgasm problem reflects on me."

- She believes that "his erection problem reflects on me."

Also, whether young or old, gay or straight, male or female, when American adults have sex, they frequently:

- Are self-conscious or self-critical about their body

- Don't feel as close to their partner as they'd like

- Don't feel confident that they're going to have a good time (which is why they don't do it more frequently)

- Are concerned about performance—either their own or their partner's

- Feel inhibited about communicating what they want, don't want, feel, or don't feel

Health problems are also frequently part of "normal" sex—because normal people have health problems.

So, are you starting to look pretty "normal"? Are you starting to realize this might not be the right goal?

I want to change things for you—and not by improving your "sexual function." This book isn't literary Viagra. It's more like literary brain surgery (sorry, no tummy tuck, boob job, or hair implants, just brain surgery).

The awkwardness and emotional isolation described above are what most people get when they try to have "normal" sex. And that's why your vision of sex matters.

So let's spend the rest of the chapter exploring why it's not important to be sexually "normal" and why, in fact, pursuing "normal" sex is often destructive.

Of course, by "normal" sex most people don't mean the reality I've just described, but a romanticized vision of perfect performance, perfect environment, and nothing too novel or psychologically challenging. The only thing normal about that kind of sex is the fact that so many people aspire to it, and so few people have it. (And here's a secret every sex therapist knows: even when people get this kind of sex, they're not necessarily satisfied with it.)

So if, like so many other people, you've been pursuing the wrong thing ("normal" sex), you need a new way to think about sex. Although most people assume it's logical to have a performance orientation (how many times per week, how many minutes before orgasm), that's only one way to look at sex. And it's exactly the wrong way.

Normality Anxiety

Most people really, really don't want to be sexually "abnormal."

So they hide sexual aspects of themselves they think might be abnormal. They focus on things they think are normal, even if they aren't that interesting. Sooner or later, this self-censorship and pretend-wholesomeness usually causes problems—because of the secrecy, the anxiety, the self-criticism, and the boredom.

It doesn't matter what in particular you think is sexually normal and abnormal. If you're concerned about this, if this concern shapes your behavior, your fantasies, or what you share with a partner, it's almost certainly undermining your sexual pleasure and closeness.

I want to rescue you from that. Not by persuading you that you're sexually "normal," but by persuading you to not care.

The Two Sides of "Normal" Sex

Americans generally think of "normal" sex as having two components—a practical one and a less tangible, "moral" one.

The Practical Side of "Normal" Sex

Most people define "normal" sex with reference to what the bodies do, particularly the genitals (penis, vagina, vulva) and the mouth.

Physicians, therapists, and drug companies use language that supports this approach. Both professionals and popular advertising talk about "function" and "dysfunction." Clinicians talk about what's normal and what's pathological. We talk about "sex" when we mean intercourse. We talk about "intimacy" and "romance" when we mean sex.

The physical side of so-called normal sex is the trajectory of desire, arousal, excitement, and orgasm. This reflects the model developed by Masters and Johnson in the 1960s, which we'll examine more closely in Chapter 4. People unconsciously use this model when they use the word *foreplay,* by which they generally mean "stuff we do before real sex—i.e., intercourse."

Most Americans categorize sexual activities as either intercourse ("real sex") or foreplay; anything else is generally considered mere fooling around or flirting—or just plain perverse. The conventional idea is that all sexual activity is supposed to culminate in intercourse, and that it's usually clear if a kiss or caress is foreplay or not. "Settling" for foreplay if a couple has the option of "real sex" isn't considered normal.

There's a small group of sexual activities on which there's a positive "normality" consensus. Intercourse and open-mouth kissing (and, please note, *only* these) are pretty universally accepted among Americans. Oral sex is now considered normal by a majority of (but not nearly all) adults, followed by hand-on-partner's-genitals. Vibrator-on-vulva is making a strong move toward normality this decade (especially among the young and well-educated), although vibrator-on-penis or vibrator-in-anus aren't even close. In fact anything with the anus is generally disqualified. Role-playing, S/M, fetishes—few people think they're normal. Most people don't even think they're "sex." So there's a majority "normality" consensus about these things, too—they aren't.

So, to do normal sex, people need to have certain body parts behaving in "normal" ways—erection on demand, plenty of vaginal lubrication on demand, etc. Of course, clinicians know that our genitalia are particularly susceptible to various common influences: emotions, stress, alcohol, disease, fatigue, even longevity of relationship. Thus, these body parts may not behave as we wish; interestingly, many people don't want to acknowledge this.

That's why a lot of my work is with people whose bodies fail to act "normal" under circumstances that *they* think are normal; my job is to convince them to get away from this destructive model, so hard to achieve in real life. Maybe you're reading this book because you're familiar with the feeling that your body has "failed" you.

So interestingly enough, while most people think taking Viagra to deal with erection problems is normal, most people think the same person using a strap-on dildo for the same reason is abnormal. Similarly, many people think a menopausal woman using hormones to increase vaginal lubrication is normal, but many people would consider her abnormal if she was using fantasy or porn for the same purpose.

The Moral Aspect of "Normal" Sex

Once we move beyond how bodies are supposed to behave during sex, and which activities qualify, it's much harder to figure out what makes for "normal" sex. Are fantasies a part of "normal" sex? How about games? Or toys? What kinds of experimentation qualify? And what about preferences—say, for masturbation over partner sex, or for oral sex over intercourse? Most people can say what *isn't* normal—but they have trouble saying why, or what rules they use to decide.

Sometimes even two partners can't agree on this. You can imagine the problems caused when one partner tells the other, "What you want us to do in bed isn't normal." That's so much worse than "No thank you."

So one way to approach this issue is to ask: what's the opposite of "normal" sex?

When I ask patients this question, both men and women typically answer with words like *kinky, perverse, dangerous, violent, immoral, out of control, unusual,* and *hedonistic.* Occasionally I get *satanic,* which makes for an interesting conversation.

Most people have an intuitive sense of what's sexually normal and what isn't. But unless we just mean "statistically common," it's virtually impossible to define precisely what we *mean* by sexually normal. Psychologists and even sex therapists disagree among themselves about it.

That said, it's especially interesting that most descriptions of normal and abnormal sex ultimately focus on two issues—control and corruption.

Even when people disagree about their standards—Joe thinks a blindfold and handcuffs are normal but a whip isn't, while his best friend thinks "all that stuff is just too kinky for words"—we're typically referring to the same ideas: boundaries and contamination.

"Normal" is an attempt to establish boundaries around sex so it can't escape, acquire too much power, or hurt others. "Normal" is an attempt to make sex small enough that it doesn't threaten us or even require us to grow. "Normal" is a recognition that eroticism resides in the unconscious, an untidy little junkyard if ever there was one.

What, for example, would you do if you found yourself enjoying something you believed was sexually abnormal? Would you change your mind about the sex, or about yourself? Or would you laugh the whole thing off and try to forget it?

I see examples of this in my practice all the time. Take Arthur, who discovered during masturbation that he gets really excited from a light stroking of his perineum (the surface between the anus and the back of the scrotum). Once he decided it was "too gay," however, he never did it again. Or take Serena: she doesn't like to have her breasts squeezed much at all, but once she's turned on she loves to have her nipples pulled and bitten—in fact, she used to climax this way before a lover told her it was "really, really weird." And she believed him.

Arthur and Serena came to see me together for couples counseling, each with several such sexual secrets. And although they'd been partners for three years, neither had revealed what they knew about their own arousal patterns; in fact, both of them deliberately stayed away from the stimulation they felt was abnormal. Talking about these things was terrifying for them—and liberating. They ended up learning much more about each other—and themselves—than they ever expected.

Our obsession with "normal" is an attempt to stay clean while dealing with something potentially dirty.

Partly because sex deals with body fluids, partly because it deals with execretory organs (literally or in the neighborhood), partly because it deals with the mysteries of pregnancy and birth, partly because it's just damn messy, and partly because sex can release us from the normal rules of physical respectability and restraint, it's often seen as something to engage in from a certain psychic distance.

Is smelling a lover's underwear normal? What about asking him or her to wear the same pair for days at a time, then smelling them? What about oral sex during menstruation? Or swallowing semen? Or *loving* to swallow semen? What about tongue-kissing first thing in the morning, when you have dragon-breath?

What's important is not whether a specific activity is or isn't normal. What's important is the concept of "normal" sex itself. As long as some things are normal, there will, by definition, be things that are abnormal. And if you don't want to think of yourself as sexually abnormal, that ultimately requires eternal vigilance. But no one can fully enjoy sex under that oppressive regime.

Cultural Norms

American ideas of what's sexually normal have changed dramatically in just the last sixty years.

In 1948 America was scandalized when Dr. Alfred Kinsey's research showed that a substantial number of American couples were practicing cunnilingus. Now marriage counselors encourage it.

Before 1965 contraception was illegal in the United States (until *Griswold v. Connecticut*), and until 1972 it was illegal for unmarried people (*Baird v. Eisenstadt*). Until 1967 sex with someone of a different race was illegal (*Loving v. Virginia*). And non-intercourse sex (sodomy) was only decriminalized in 2003 (*Lawrence v. Texas*). That's a lot of change in a very short time.

Ideas of what's sexually normal are dramatically different from country to country, too. In China, for example, adults generally don't kiss in public; even holding hands is considered risqué. In

most of Europe, adults and children typically go to the beach top-
less or nude. (They don't consider this a sexual practice, but that's
the point—in America we do.) Clitoridectomy (female genital cutting) is practiced by Muslims in North Africa, the Middle East, and
Southeast Asia on about two million girls each year; in the United
States it's illegal and considered violent child abuse. Premarital sex
is expected and considered normal in Holland and Scandinavia,
where sexual decision-making is freely discussed within families.

Each new advance in technology raises the issue of sexual normality all over again. Here are just a few recent American examples:

- *Videocassette recorders:* Between 1980 and 1990, over two-
  thirds of American TV households acquired a VCR. This
  phenomenal rise in consumer interest was driven to a large
  extent by the new chance to watch pornography privately.
  But was watching porn "normal"? And what kind of porn?
  Should a husband hide his porn-watching from his wife?
  Should he invite her to join him? Should she accept?

- *The Internet:* When cheap, high-speed broadband hit
  America in 2000, tens of millions of people immediately
  became involved in "virtual relationships," either as
  themselves or via representations. Second Life, chat rooms,
  instant messaging, phone sex, age play, gender play, role
  play—the opportunities are now literally endless. Suddenly
  people are coming into contact with sexual subcultures,
  ideas, and behaviors that just a short while ago were
  completely invisible to them. And now many people are
  wondering: Is it normal, kinky, or downright sick for an
  adult to pretend to be a teen, a millionaire, a spy, the other
  gender? How many hours a week (or day!) is it okay to spend
  on the Internet in these pursuits? Is sexy chat with a stranger
  a form of infidelity, a sign of insecurity, a new frontier of
  eroticism? Perhaps all three? Law enforcement demands that
  people stop age play, claiming it encourages child molesting.
  While they have no data to support this claim, state and
  federal governments now spend tens of millions of dollars in

precious tax money stalking and entrapping those interested in age play with other adults.

- *Cell phones/sexting:* Three-quarters of teens have cell phones, and millions of them are "sexting"—sending or receiving sexually explicit photos of themselves and their peers. Law enforcement has gotten heavily involved, attempting to wipe out the activity with the claim that it's terribly dangerous, demanding enormous penalties—felony jail time and sex offender registration. Parents are trapped in between. They tend to feel it's more harmful than kids do, but less dangerous—and less worthy of draconian punishment— than legislators and law enforcement do.

In each of these cases, the question "what is sexually normal?" is of great interest socially, politically, and economically. There is still no consensus on any of these fronts, which shows that whatever we come to believe is sexually "normal" is culturally negotiated, not inevitable or somehow "natural."

Ten years ago, who would have thought that any of the following would be considered as mainstream ("normal") as they are today?

- Erotic spanking, blindfolding, and handcuffing

- Vibrators (now available on Amazon.com)

- Swing clubs

- Internet pornography

- Hotel room pay-for-pornography

- Coarse language on HBO and basic cable TV

Once you realize that what you think you know about "normal" sex is just one idea among many, a whole world of eroticism will open to you. A sexual world beyond self-criticism and anxiety, be-yond orgasm, beyond success and failure. And that's where sexual relaxation, enjoyment, and intimacy can truly take place.

Why Is Focusing on Normality a Problem?

The fact is, anxiety about being sexually normal creates emotional isolation. That's why many people are at their loneliest when they're making love.

For most people, emotional isolation kills genuine sexual desire and pleasure.

Focusing on "normal" sexuality makes sex an enterprise with stakes that are too high. At any moment, our preferences, fantasies, or inhibitions can expose us as unacceptable—to ourselves or to our partner. Being "normal" (in other words, not abnormal) becomes more important than feeling pleasure or closeness. Fearing judgment, we don't do the things we'd do if we didn't fear being judged (for example, a man asking to have his nipples pulled). And we do things we otherwise wouldn't (such as intercourse when we're not ready) if we didn't imagine that that's what normal people do.

So our yearning to be sexually normal, combined with our anxiety that we aren't, leads us to keep sexual secrets from our partner. Being authentic appears to involve just too much of a gamble.

Neither pleasure nor intimacy can flourish in such an environment. In this setting, a lost erection is a disaster. Difficulty climaxing is a crisis. Farting or wetting the bed is a tragedy.

And not just for one person, but for his or her partner too. Because many people focus not only on their own "function" but on their partner's too—and they take their partner's functioning personally. Many people scrutinize their partner's arousal and orgasm because they don't want to be judged a failure—a "poor lover." But how can you relax when your partner is examining your sexual response—not in a joyful, attentive way, but with an eye for signs that he or she has failed?

———————

Jedd was a gruff-looking, gruff-talking guy, an electrician whose hands looked like they'd been earning a living for years.

Within minutes of sitting down, he told me three things: he grew up in a poor Italian family in Brooklyn, he loved his wife Martina, and he was wearing pantyhose. Apparently, those facts were of roughly equal importance. Guess which one he and Martina had been fighting about?

It had started a few years before with panties—hers. When she found out ("More and more of them were getting stretched out, and I couldn't understand why. Then I figured it out"), he gave her a book to read on the subject, and they had a long talk. He made it clear he wasn't gay. "I believed him then, and I believe him now," she said.

Like most straight men who wear women's underwear, he liked the feel. And it helped him relax. But he couldn't just enjoy his little hobby. He wanted to discuss it with Martina. "Constantly," she said. "It was always, 'I want to make sure you understand. I want to make sure you know I'm not sick. I want it to be okay with you, and not something we have to hide.' We had to talk about it every day."

"See, you really don't like it!" Jedd was almost triumphant.

Martina turned to me. "I don't care that he wears panties, or stockings, or any damn thing," she sighed. "He buys his own stuff, he keeps it with his clothes, I don't care. Can we please change the subject? I'd like to go a whole week without talking about it. I'd like to have my husband back!"

"Doc, she thinks I'm weird. Tell her I'm not." Before I could speak, Martina jumped in. "Of course I think it's weird," she growled. "But so what? You're not perfect, Jedd, and frankly, there are other things you do that bother me a lot more."

Jedd was clear. "We can't get our sex life back until you accept this about me." Martina looked at me, really frustrated. "In Brooklyn, in the old days, we knew that the only way to deal with a person this stubborn would be to just kill them." We all smiled.

"Jedd, how do *you* feel about dressing like this?" I asked. "There's nothing wrong with it," he replied defiantly. "Jedd, I'm a sex therapist," I said. "You're not the first guy I ever met who wears pantyhose. My question is, how do *you* feel about it?"

"There's nothing wrong with it," he said softly. He repeated it, with tears in his eyes. He'd been saying it—to his wife, to himself—for years, but he didn't really believe it. He was ashamed of what he liked, and ashamed of what he was doing.

"It's hard to believe that Martina accepts it when you don't, isn't it?" I gently asked. "You know she's upset about how much you *talk* about it, not how much you *do* it, right?" He nodded. "And maybe if *you* accepted it a little more, you wouldn't have to talk about it so much, right?" Again a nod.

In truth, neither of them was wild about Jedd's interest in women's underwear. He didn't quite understand why he was so drawn to it, and she didn't understand why he was so adamant about the whole thing, alternately demanding and pleading for acceptance.

"Jedd, talking about this all the time is driving Martina crazy," I said. "That doesn't mean she rejects you. Any subject gets boring if you talk about it too much, whether it's lasagna or Notre Dame football or Jedd-wearing-panties.

"But if you're talking about it this much, you must be concerned about it, right?"

Yes, he said, he had concerns he needed to talk about. "Ordinarily, you'd talk with a friend, or Martina's brother, maybe even a priest," I ventured.

"Forget all of them," he laughed.

"Right. Then maybe you should see your own individual thera-pist about this," I suggested.

"I don't want a shrink to tell me I'm crazy," said Jedd.

"No, you want someone to talk to, right?" And I referred him to someone knowledgeable with whom he could talk.

"Once you're seeing him," I said, "I'd like you to limit your conversations with Martina about this—at least for a little while, okay?" Martina was delighted, but concerned. "Jedd, we'll still talk about all the other things we always talk about, right?"

"And maybe, Jedd, when you've come to terms with your inter-ests, you can relax enough to have sex with Martina again," I said matter-of-factly.

"Yes," said the tough guy from Brooklyn. "I admit that she's been here all along for me. I want to be her man again."

Lies, Damned Lies, and Statistics

Every week, couples in conflict ask me what's sexually normal. Is sex once per month during the first year of marriage normal? Is getting turned on by spanking—or being spanked—normal? How long should intercourse last before the guy ejaculates? Is wanting oral sex during menstruation normal? Is getting turned off by nasty talk normal?

Sometimes people are worried about themselves. Sometimes they're critical of their partner, and they want to wheel in the heavy artillery of "You're not normal. *I'm* normal."

Every year around Valentine's Day I get the same kind of ques-tions from the popular media. And although I know the current statistics—how many times per month, how many inches, how many minutes—I generally don't mention these, whether I'm talk-ing to patients or to *USA Today* (the newspaper delivered free to your hotel room so you have something to read while brushing your teeth). I say that deliberately or not, people generally make trouble with these numbers, and they're better off without them.

Nobody is satisfied with this answer.

I say forget the number of times people have sex per month, or how often someone masturbates, or how long it takes to climax. Those averages tell you nothing. Knowing that you don't laugh during sex, are too embarrassed to use lubricant, or can't tell your partner, "No, not there, here," tells us much, much more.

Because that describes your experience. And that's what sex is about—experience, not numbers. What really matters in sex isn't the things you can measure; it's how people *feel*, which is a lot harder to explore, understand, measure, or fix. And as with all problems, if you're trying to fix the wrong thing, it doesn't matter what you accomplish.

That's why, when it comes to sex, conventional self-help usually doesn't help, because it generally doesn't challenge people's basic ideas about what "normal" sex is. More importantly, how could self-help help when it doesn't challenge the idea that it's important to be sexually "normal," and *very* important to not be sexually abnormal?

Instead, most self-help books are *prescriptive*: they tell people exactly what kind of sex they *should* have, and then tell them how to have it. That approach obviously hasn't worked very well. That's why people are still buying self-help books, still going to sex therapy, still begging *The View* to feature yet more "sexperts."

What every self-help book and guru needs to say is that people's desire to be sexually normal keeps them from being their authentic sexual selves, leading to performance anxiety and sexual dissatisfaction. Sexual Intelligence—based on self-knowledge, self-acceptance, and profound communication—is a better approach to resolving sexual dissatisfaction.

If you want to know what's sexually normal, remember these features:

Chapter Three

What Is Sexual Intelligence? Why Does It Matter?

I started seeing Margot and Duane a year after their first child was born. They were pretty upset that they had stopped having sex regularly. They couldn't figure out why one or both of them always had an excuse.

The two thirty-two-year-olds had most of what society thinks people need for great sex: They were both drop-dead gorgeous. Duane made a lot of money. They had paid help with child care. They not only loved each other, they seemed to like each other, too. So why no sex? Or as Margot put it, "Why do we have this desire dysfunction?"

Asking a lot of questions during a series of sessions, I got to know them pretty well. As with most of my patients, we uncovered some pretty strong reasons for the behavior they said they wanted to change. And no, neither of them had a "dysfunction."

In fact, Margot really loved sex—and loved it with Duane. Unlike some women who have little interest in sex after a day alone with an active, healthy infant, Margot wanted her husband to lust after her. She said she "needed" this in order to feel appreciated, adult, and sexy—which she didn't especially feel after finger-painting all day. She was absolutely ready to respond to practically any sexual invitation—which kept not coming.

Duane loved sex too, and loved it with Margot. But after working a twelve-hour day and putting his daughter to sleep soon after he got home, he could barely keep his eyes open. He yearned to tumble into bed with his sexy wife—and have her supply the energy for their erotic life. But no matter how much she talked about sex, or envied other sexy-looking couples, she never initiated.

Of course, they didn't have this problem in the good old days. When they were courting just out of college, they would have sex every morning and every night. They both clearly remembered that no one initiated sex back then—it would "just happen." And they were each waiting for it to "just happen" again. That's not a "dysfunction"—it's just an unfortunate idea.

We discussed their wish for sex to be as it was when they were younger. I explained that their lives had changed and that, for sex to "happen," someone would have to initiate. Yes, that person might hear the word "no"; they were both stunned to even imagine such a thing, since the idea was so different from the sexual era they remembered. And, even if they were to resume having sex, their encounters probably wouldn't be for an hour or two like they used to be. That prospect wasn't really acceptable to them either.

They kept insisting that they loved sex and wanted sex—but they didn't want the sex I suggested was available to them. So they continued having no sex, wondering how things could change.

Meanwhile, Margot was ready to conceive again as soon as possible. After all, she really, really, *really* wanted a son.

And so, with Marilyn already almost two, it was time for the second one.

Duane wasn't so eager. And that didn't help their sex life. As I told them, "Working on a sexual relationship while dealing with fertility questions is like trying to rotate your tires while driving seventy miles per hour on the freeway."

Nevertheless, they wanted to continue working with me, and I agreed. For his own reasons, Duane soon agreed to try for a son, telling Margot only one thing: "I'm concerned about what will happen if we don't have a son. I don't want to keep trying endlessly, okay?" Only slightly troubled, she happily said yes. They conceived almost immediately—no "dysfunction" there.

They took a break from therapy once Margot was a few months pregnant. Right on schedule, they finally had that second child, a beautiful, healthy girl.

Five months after little Charlotte was born, Duane and Margot were back in my office. Many women take as long as a year after giving birth before recovering their sexual desire. Not Margot—three weeks after having their daughter, she was ready for sex. Announcing this to Duane, she resumed waiting for him to chase her around the house.

Of course, Margot felt very apologetic about her body— she was still ten pounds more than her pre-pregnancy weight, and her personal grooming wasn't quite back up to her usual rigorous standards. So she wanted sex, but she also wanted advance notice so she could wax, bathe, tweeze, use her lotions, and so on. This made sex even more complicated.

Duane, too, hesitated to resume sex—for completely different reasons. He scoffed at Margot's suggestion that her beautiful body was less desirable than it had been. But he did admit that birth control was very much on his mind. He was happy with his two kids, son or no son. He already felt overwhelmed, and believed she did, too. But he feared she'd be devastated if he explicitly refused to try for a son, so he didn't talk about it seriously enough for Margot to really hear it.

She needed to be chased, and so couldn't initiate; he was anxious about being pushed to try for a son (and becoming accidentally pregnant), so he couldn't initiate. And so month after month, they'd been skipping the great sex they remembered having years before.

Neither of them wanted to use condoms (she thought them "yucky," he thought them unreliable). She didn't want to use hormonal methods like the pill because of possible side effects or weight gain.

They talked about whether Margot could ever be happy with "just" two wonderful, healthy daughters. She said she didn't need a son right away, and maybe, maybe could even live without one. But she couldn't decide that now.

Meanwhile, they weren't having sex. She wanted him to initiate, and he didn't want to risk another pregnancy.

And so I asked about sex without any risk of conceiving—outercourse. Oral sex, anal play, hands-on-genitals, biting, whispering, sucking, stroking, playing. "Oh, foreplay," Margot said dismissively. "I'd rather have sex."

"We used to do all that stuff," Duane said. And now? "Well, I love Margot's blow jobs, but then we both want sex afterwards. And I'd feel guilty if I got a great blow job and Margot was still frustrated about not having real sex."

The only dysfunction here was their distorted beliefs about "real sex." Their mutual resistance to great-sex-without-intercourse was fascinating: it wasn't "real sex," it wasn't their favorite kind, it was kinda dumb, they shouldn't "need to" do it, they'd feel silly doing this second-rate thing. The usual explanations I hear every week.

It was a massive failure of imagination—and a demonstration of their limited Sexual Intelligence. "We know what great sex looks like—we used to have it all the time. And that stuff isn't it," Margot pouted. Agreeing, Duane predicted that "just outercourse" would leave them emotionally hungry. So they continued not having sex at all, emotionally starving and needing more emotional connection.

I tried to dig deeper to understand what all this resistance was about.

"First you say sex will never be like it used to be, then you say we shouldn't expect to have real sex until we solve the question of another child," said a frustrated Margot. "To accept this, I'd, I'd, I'd . . . have to change!" she sputtered.

"Yes," I nodded sympathetically. "If you and your husband want to have sex at this stage in your lives, you'll have to change." They said they were on board. But no matter how I discussed it, they just couldn't adjust to the idea. And so these bright, attractive, horny people rejected sex again.

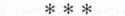

The Value of Intelligence

We just saw how one couple pushed sex away because it couldn't provide a particular kind of validation. We've looked at how people attempt to get this relief and reassurance—mostly by pursuing superb genital function. This is supposed to give you mythologically huge orgasms and lead to your partner's rapturous satisfaction.

Rather than talk about how to enhance genital function, let's turn instead to an entirely different way of thinking about sex. Let's talk about what you actually need to create and sustain sexual pleasure and closeness over time. As a bonus, this approach will also provide relief from self-consciousness and self-criticism, and dramatically reduce your need for reassurance about your sexual normality and adequacy.

This different approach involves developing and using your Sexual Intelligence. Sexual Intelligence is the set of internal resources that allows you to relax, be present, communicate, respond to stimulation, and create physical and emotional connection with a partner. When you can do that, you'll have enjoyable sexual experiences, regardless of what your body does. Compared to that kind of emotional and physical nourishment, the biggest, hardest erection or the wettest, tightest vagina are trivial.

Sexual Intelligence is more than knowledge, more than patience, more than confidence, and more than liking your own body. It's all of these, but it's more.

"Intelligence," of course, is a familiar and useful concept. It can be defined by ability: the ability to learn or to solve problems. It can be defined narrowly: as innate cognitive capacity or the facility for abstract thought, and it can be defined broadly: as the ability to understand different ways of learning and organizing information and to select the best one in a given situation.

Imagine waking up tomorrow, completely by surprise and unprepared, in Moscow. You don't speak Russian, and you have only your passport and 3,000 rubles. (Let's say it's summertime—we don't want you freezing before completing the thought-experiment.) To figure out what to do, you would need more than *knowledge*—you would need *intelligence*. You'd need the ability to figure out what questions to ask, how to find people who can help you, how to make decisions in a different culture, and so on.

That's what Sexual Intelligence is like—not the ability to be great in bed, or to function the way you did when you were twenty-two. Rather, Sexual Intelligence is expressed in the ability to create and maintain desire in a situation that's less than perfect or comfortable; the capacity to adapt to your changing body; curiosity and open-mindedness about the meaning of pleasure, closeness, and satisfaction; and the ability to adjust when things don't go as expected—when you run out of lube, or one of you has to go to the bathroom during sex, or you lose your erection, or one of you calls the other by the wrong name. Or all of these at the same time. (There's a Will Farrell movie in there somewhere.)

That's why everyone needs Sexual Intelligence. And that's why with it, you can relax and enjoy sex in ways you may have thought impossible for you.

To manage their anxiety, their sexuality, and their partner's sexuality, most people rely on the usual ways of looking at sexuality: "normal" sex, genital function and "dysfunction," self-monitoring, trying to remember "what women want," and so on. Most of my patients (and you, perhaps?) have proven that this limited approach doesn't lead to pleasure and closeness. What do they need instead? Not technique or a great body, but Sexual Intelligence.

So what exactly is this Sexual Intelligence?

The Three Components of Sexual Intelligence

The three components of Sexual Intelligence are:

1. Information and knowledge

2. Emotional skills (which let you use that knowledge)

3. Body awareness and comfort (which let you express yourself and your knowledge)

The *knowledge* that most people seem to want about sex is "how can I be great in bed?" For those with a conventional "dysfunction," the question usually takes the form: "How can I function right?

How can I get rid of my dysfunction?" (This always sounds to me like: "How can I get my penis or vulva to sit up and do tricks?")

In addition, many people ask me: "How can I get my partner to be more skillful or enthusiastic in bed?" "What do men/women really want during sex?" and "What positions give the most satisfaction?"

Although I sympathize with people's wish to be (or feel) more sexually competent, I think that's the wrong goal. Answering questions like these is *not* an effective path to creating more enjoyable sex.

No, the information you actually need would start with a uniquely personal owner's manual to your body and your partner's body, including your preferences (and your partner's) about touching and kissing. Ideally, this manual would include the kinds of bodily changes you could expect over time—changes in the consistency of vaginal lubrication, the effect of hormonal changes on your sexual response, and so on. A reminder that back pain or a stiff shoulder greatly influences sex would also help.

An anthropologist's field report on the incredible diversity of human sexuality would be valuable too. It would help put your (and your partner's) experiences, fantasies, preferences, and curiosity in context, reducing your anxiety about normality.

A lot of what you need for more enjoyable sex isn't specifically sexual. *Emotional skills* are necessary for satisfaction in many aspects of life, including sex. There is, to put it simply, no substitute for growing up—not even a perfect body or the best sexual technique. It's like trying to run a car by stuffing hundred-dollar bills into the gas tank. The money itself won't make the car run; it's only of value if you can first convert it to gasoline. Emotional skills are the gasoline of enjoyable sex.

If people wanted only physical pleasure from sex, we could make the argument that only physical skills and knowledge are relevant. (I wouldn't make that argument, but sooner or later someone on daytime TV would.) As we've seen, however, most women and men want more than physical pleasure from sex. So it makes perfect sense that we need emotional skills to create those other satisfactions. After all, how many times would you want to make love with someone—no matter how good-looking or talented—who was rude, self-involved, scared of closeness, and a terrible listener? (No ex-husband jokes here, please.)

Finally, we come to *the body*—the actual location of all that huffing and puffing we call sex. The popular idea of the body's role in sex is that it should be beautiful, the better to trigger desire in both a partner and ourselves (as if looking in the mirror is what turns us on). This idea explains why so many people don't feel sexy, and why they assume they aren't sexy to others. And it makes people feel less eligible for sex as they get older.

Furthermore, it's the body that supposedly does the exotic, athletic things that produce pleasure in ourselves and our partner.

Of course, this means that the body has to "function correctly." Back in 1966, researchers William Masters and Virginia Johnson defined the Sexual Response Cycle—the standard way human bodies respond to sexual stimulation. Everyone immediately compared themselves to this model; for those who missed it, *Cosmopolitan* and *Playboy* issued plenty of impractical, improbable instructions in the 1970s and 1980s. After that, Oprah and Dr. Phil spent two uptight decades telling everyone exactly what was sexually right and normal (i.e., what was sexually wrong and abnormal). Now, of course, everyone has pornography to provide unrealistic images of bodies during sex.

This book's idea is different. Let's view the body as a vehicle for attunement with a partner, and let's enhance your body's tolerance for pleasure and intensity. Let's make sure your body is responding to what's present during sex, rather than having semi-traumatized reactions to old aggravating or painful experiences.

These perspectives are all more important than "functioning" or beauty or athleticism or technique. Besides, you can't talk your body into functioning a certain way just by trying hard.

Together, the three aspects of Sexual Intelligence are what let our eroticism flow. They *support* functioning without putting functioning in the center of our sexual thinking or experience. When people say they want sex to be more "intimate," they're actually referring to aspects of Sexual Intelligence, such as self-acceptance, trust, good boundaries, and self-knowledge (all of which we'll examine in Part Two).

What's *not* included in Sexual Intelligence are things such as physical stamina, lots of sexual experience, youth, and the Timeless Techniques of the Mystic Orient. Yes, even though the media and their "sexperts" claim that physical qualities and special techniques are what create "great sex," they are not the way to create the sexual experiences that *you want*.

Take, for example, Josip and Renata.

What do you get when you put two lawyers in the same marriage?

The serious answer is, "It all depends"; in Josip and Renata's case, it was trouble. They just couldn't get away from their adversarial approach to each other.

It would be easy to blame their professional backgrounds for this, but that wouldn't be accurate. These were two people who had difficulty trusting anyone. Being lawyers just enabled them to make a living out of their personality deficits.

At home, meanwhile, they quarreled a lot: low-level bickering that periodically burst into yelling, blaming, and name-calling. They'd regret doing it in front of their kids, try to understand how things got out of hand, fail, promise to try harder, and get ready for the next round.

Why did they come to see me? They wanted to have sex more often, and they wanted to enjoy it more.

At this point you might be shaking your head—how do people expect to enjoy sex under these circumstances? And yet this is pretty common—people living in a less-than-perfect relationship wanting to have good sex. Unfortunately, there are no time-outs in life, so people can't escape their marriages (or their emotional problems) while trying to improve their sex lives.

Since Josip and Renata were not hesitant to fight in front of me, I became familiar with their dynamic pretty quickly. They'd talk about some disappointment or frustration at home—him being late for dinner, her obsessing about the kids' safety—and although they'd try to discuss things calmly, they quickly escalated. Within a minute or two, they'd be fighting about how "you always do this" and "you never do that."

We really needed to do Marriage Counseling 101, which Renata hated. "I'm not a dummy, and I won't be lectured to. I know how to be married," she declared. Josip tried to calm her. "I think it would be great if we understood ourselves better," he offered. "Especially you."

You go help these people with their sex lives.

I explained that before we talked about orgasms, caressing, or positions, we needed to improve their ability to tolerate closeness with each other. They agreed that would be "nice," although they really wanted to focus more on sex. "If we had more sex, maybe we wouldn't fight as much," Josip suggested. "Yes," said Renata. "After Josip climaxes, he's nice to me for hours, sometimes even for the next day or two."

Realizing they were not going to be deterred from their ideas about sex and intimacy, I replied that I supported them in having enjoyable sex. "And I'm certain it will help," I continued, "if you each learn these five skills":

- Comforting yourself when frustrated

- Giving your mate the benefit of the doubt

- When hurt, redefining the other person as uninformed rather than uncaring

- Imagining how you sound to your mate before you say something

- Striving to understand your mate before striving to be understood

"I agree that Josip needs to grow up," Renata said sharply. "But this all sounds like psychoanalysis. And besides, I don't need to learn these things. I need for my husband to spend more time with me, and to not be such a jerk."

Josip tried to respond cooperatively, but within minutes they were both being loudly sarcastic, each blaming the other for not trying harder to be sexy. Every mean thing they said just proved my point. Then I got an idea.

"Okay, you want a specifically sexual exercise. This week at home, I'd like you to do the hand massage as described in this handout* I'm giving you. Will you agree?" "Oh finally, something about sex," Renata said, taking the form I offered. Scanning it quickly, she wrinkled her nose. "It's just about hands," she complained. "Well, it's about bodies and pleasure," I replied, familiar with that response after assigning this homework to a hundred couples over the years.

They said they'd do it.

The next week, they reported they hadn't. "She fought with me most of the week," Josip said. "Including the one time we sat down to do the stupid homework," Renata added. I didn't say a word, and the room fell silent for a few moments. "Okay, maybe we should talk more about how to get along better," she sighed.

We're still working on it.

---

*Reproduced on page 241.

This couple keeps wanting to know when we're going to talk about sex. I keep focusing on enhancing their ability to trust, be patient, exercise self-discipline, and see each other as friends—in short, making their relationship one in which a sexual connection would make sense. That's a key aspect of Sexual Intelligence—enhancing the relationship to enhance the sex. Some people think it works in the opposite direction. It almost never does.

Sexual Intelligence as a Narrative

Everybody tells stories about themselves. I don't just mean "Where did you buy that car?" or "What's your favorite TV show?" We're *always* telling other people about who we are, always relying on some narrative to explain ourselves—big-picture stories, descriptions of what's important, who we are, and how we got to be that person.

When it comes to sex, each of us also has a narrative. These narratives answer fundamental questions about our identity: When it comes to sex, who are you? Why? How did you get that way? Here are some common narratives about sexuality: *I am . . .*

☐ scared of sex

☐ impulsive, a risk-taker

☐ a romantic

☐ always horny

☐ undersexed

☐ oversexed

☐ always ready for more

☐ unlucky with men/women

☐ no good at sex

☐ good in bed

☐ still getting over my last experience

☐ unable to communicate my needs

☐ frightened of men/women

☐ not sexually desirable

☐ not good at trust

☐ done with sex

☐ interested in lovemaking, not "sex"

☐ a victim of date rape or childhood sexual exploitation

☐ confused about the whole sex thing

☐ a sucker for a good line

☐ a sex addict

As an organizing principle for thinking about sex, Sexual Intelligence is a kind of narrative: of personal adequacy, of presence, of connection, of sufficiency, of agency and ownership of your own body, of relaxation (whether you're excited or not), and of acceptance (of things as they are rather than as you imagine or fear them).

Sexual Intelligence is also a narrative of *not* caring about what isn't important. Of course, first you have to decide what that is. Then you need the self-discipline to ignore it, even when others value it and it seems to beckon you.

Here are some things my patients pay attention to during sex (or between sexual encounters) that interfere with their sexual enjoyment:

- The desire and ability to do *every* sexual thing

- Who's hurt them before

- Feeling competitive with all men/women or with their partner's previous partner(s)

- Conventional "distractions" (undone chores, the sound of the TV in another part of the house)

I work with my patients to decide that these things aren't important, and I help them develop the self-discipline to ignore them. Many people don't realize the role of self-discipline in creating enjoyable sex—and in enjoying it. Perhaps you picture good sex as wild and carefree (which of course it can be), and assume that it's therefore completely spontaneous and free of boundaries. But that's like imagining that an enjoyable meal or a nice day in the park just happens without any preparation or mental focus. If you've ever gone to a popular bistro and spent your meal fretting about the location of your table, or gone on a picnic and obsessed about running out of sunscreen, you know that deliberately focusing your attention on what's important is a key part of enjoying activities.

The same is true for sex—to enjoy it you have to be mentally prepared, as well as know what *not* to pay attention to.

So the Sexual Intelligence narrative is about your actual experience, rather than a comparison of your performance, desire level, or fantasies with various standards ("manly," "youthful," "sexy," and so on). Instead of thinking about whether your performance is adequate or your fantasies are normal, this perspective helps you evaluate your sexuality according to your enjoyment, your connection with your partner, and your values.

The Sexual Intelligence approach involves changing your relationship with your sexuality, not simply getting your body to do better tricks. It's far less about what you *do,* and more about who you *are*—what you think, feel, believe, and want. That's why you won't find any instructions in this book about lingerie or toys or positions.

Enhancing your Sexual Intelligence is the most reliable and far-reaching way to enhance your sexual experience.

The concept of Sexual Intelligence helps explain why some people are sexually frustrated even though they don't have a "dysfunction" and their body works fine. It's because good "function" doesn't guarantee the closeness, physical attunement, and relaxation that makes sex enjoyable.

Because the Sexual Intelligence approach encourages and facili-

Part Two

Components of
Sexual Intelligence

Chapter Four

Your Brain

Information and Knowledge

I liked Jason as soon as I met him. He was brilliant—a Harvard undergraduate, now in his last year at Stanford Business School. He had a youthful mop of unkempt brown hair that wouldn't behave, and purple shoelaces—refreshing among the other buttoned-down MBA students.

"At twenty-five, I'm a miserable failure with women," he declared. In what way? "My erections are totally unreliable, and I sometimes ejaculate too quickly." How quickly? "Before the girl comes. You know how embarrassing that is?"

When I asked Jason what made these things a problem, he thought maybe I didn't understand his situation, so he told me again. "Yes, I understand," I said. "But why is it a problem if you don't get erect when you want to, and if you come before you want to?"

"I don't know how it was in your day," he started, half joking, half annoyed, "but today girls expect certain things when they go to bed with a guy. And a good, solid fuck is one of them. And that should include an orgasm."

"That sounds pretty intimidating," I said gently. "Is that how you feel?"

"Yes and no," he replied. "I don't feel so confident, but it seems like a reasonable expectation for a woman to have, doesn't it?"

"It depends on the details," I said. "If she prefers certain things, that's fine. If she doesn't know how to enjoy herself without these things, then she's setting you both up for failure."

This wasn't quite what he expected. "Maybe you can't help me," he challenged. "Maybe you don't understand young people, or women." This was my big chance to say something stupid. I didn't take it.

"Jason, I'm sure there are things I don't understand. And I want to get to know you better, so I can understand exactly what things mean to you. That said," I continued, "there are a few things about your situation that I think I do understand. And maybe, in fact, I can help you understand them better."

"Okay, go ahead," said Jason.

"First, I think you're overgeneralizing about what women want. I believe you're accurately describing several women you've met, and undoubtedly many more, but they're not even a majority, much less all women. Second, most women's orgasms ultimately result from clitoral, not vaginal stimulation. So intercourse, as enjoyable as it can be, is generally not the activity that makes them climax. Third, anxiety about getting erections makes it harder to get or keep an erection. And most rapid ejaculation comes from anxiety, not from too much pleasure or stimulation."

Before he could respond, I added, "These are not my opinions. These are facts.

"Now I do understand that intercourse has symbolic meaning for many men and women," I continued. "And I appreciate that you feel bad about not being able to have, or deliver, that symbolic meaning in the way you want to—in the way you feel is necessary. But let's separate practical value from symbolic meaning, and let's accept fact as fact.

"You believe you have to deliver a fast-happening, long-lasting erection, and you believe you have to make a woman orgasm with intercourse. And you believe you're not very good at all that, right?"

He nodded.

"Rather than try to fix your penis," I said, "I propose we give it a rest and change two other things—the way you approach sex, and the way you select your sex partners." The young man looked skeptical, but he was listening intently. "Let's reduce the pressure you feel before, during, and after sex. That will not only maximize your ability to get and keep an erection, it will make it easier to enjoy the sex you do have, whatever happens."

"And what about my partner's disappointment?" he asked.

"Back to my first two points, Jason," I reminded him. "First, look for women who like you for who you are, get to know them, and talk about sex before you start doing it together. Second, keep in mind that while many of them may want intercourse, for most of them it's not a have-to. If you want to know a particular woman's have-tos, ask. I can tell you from professional *and* personal experience," I said, "that the most common have-to a woman has about sex is that she wants the guy to be emotionally present. And if we're talking about her physical satisfaction, for most women intercourse is nice, but a hand, mouth, or vibrator on her clitoris is more likely to be the have-to."

As he thought over this major change in how he approached sex, I said one more thing. "Jason, take advantage of what I know."

He did. And after only a few more sessions, he was enjoying sex a lot more, and he said a grateful good-bye.

✳ ✳ ✳

Accurate information is absolutely essential for good decision-making. However, America's bizarre cultural ambivalence about sexuality mixes information together with gossip, opinion, superstition, and outright lies, so it's hard to know what to believe. In addition, many people have so much anxiety about sexuality that they have trouble using accurate information to make decisions. Examples include contraception and sterilization, oral and anal sex, fantasy, and masturbation.

Let's look at some information that can help you create sexual experiences that provide pleasure, bring you closer to your partner, and fit with your values.

Anatomy and Physiology

When I was first being trained as a sex educator (sometime between the invention of the wheel and the invention of the Internet), I learned about the sexual parts of the body—the "erogenous zones." You know, the genitalia, mouth, nipples, anus, and ears. Some liberals would also add the thighs, butt, and neck.

But eventually I came to realize—this idea is *so* wrong. The whole idea of dividing the body into sexual and non-sexual zones discourages erotic experimentation, overemphasizes orgasm, and encourages Normality Anxiety. And it doesn't reflect this common experience:

Although some body parts are terrifically sensitive under some conditions with some people, the same parts with someone else, in a physically uncomfortable location, when you haven't showered, or you're angry or embarrassed, won't be even slightly sensitive—and so at such moments, they're not sexual body parts after all.

On the other hand, perhaps you've had the experience of being so excited that your entire body was one big sexual organ. During those blessed moments, you have no non-sexual body parts.

There isn't *any* part of your body that can't be erotically charged. As you read this, somebody somewhere is making love with his or her elbow, knee, foot, hair, *breath*.

A little wiser than I was back in 1978, now I say there are no erogenous zones—because there are no non-erogenous zones. Call this approach Guerilla Anatomy: There are no sexual parts of the body. There's the body. There's erotic energy. The first experiences and expresses the second. Lather, rinse, repeat.

If there's any exception to this, it's the clitoris—the only organ in the human body with absolutely no purpose other than pleasure. You do know that most women only climax when this little pearl is stimulated (by a hand, a tongue, a vibrator, a pillow, running water, a turkey sandwich), right? A penis going in and out of the vagina generally misses the clitoris; since it doesn't matter by how much, it might as well be by a mile. And if you're keeping score at home:

clitoris + surrounding lips (labia) +
vaginal opening = vulva

For most women who want to climax, the vulva, not the vagina, is their best bet.

So why do people make such a fuss about the holiest of "erogenous zones," the genitalia? Two reasons:

1. The genitalia are the equipment we use to create a baby. It's the Miracle of Life angle—which most people try to avoid virtually every time they have sex their entire lives.

2. The genitalia have this cool hydraulic capacity: when the brain experiences stimulation that it codes as sexual (a

picture, a smell, a memory, a touch, an emotion, whatever), it sends a message down the spinal column to the pelvis, where the nerves instruct the blood vessels to open up and let in a small tidal wave. When tissue in the penis or vulva then gets engorged, the organ gets bigger and way more sensitive.

The Sexual Response Cycle

Here's the origin of the mental model most Americans have of sex. Understanding this will help you realize both the limits of how you conceptualize your body's sexual function and the value of Sexual Intelligence—an entirely different way to think about it.

In the 1960s, William Masters and Virginia Johnson studied how people's bodies function during sex—which had never been done systematically before. (Insert favorite joke here about your cousin Vinnie, who studied this for years in various cars all over Brooklyn.)

Hundreds of volunteer couples had sex in a St. Louis laboratory, while trained staff measured their skin temperature, pulse, pupil dilation, and so on. Masters and Johnson tabulated this information, which is now part of the standard training for sex therapists. They conceptualized their subjects' experience in a model they called the Sexual Response Cycle (opposite).*

The point of the model is to summarize and describe how "normal" bodies respond to "normal" stimulation. At a time when TV couldn't show married people in bed together reading or talking, and Johnny Carson wasn't allowed to say the word *pregnant* on the air, Masters and Johnson's research, and its results, were revolutionary.

---

*The multiple orgasm some women experience can also be easily drawn on this diagram. It looks like a series of waves alternating between orgasm and plateau without going all the way down to resolution.

Masters and Johnson's Sexual Response Cycle

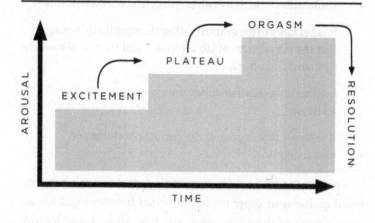

In the early 1960s, science and the machine were the dominant metaphors that Americans used in art, advertising, education, sports, and health. So that was how Masters and Johnson looked at human bodies—as machines expected to function in predictable ways. Bodies that didn't act in this predictable way had a pathology that needed to be addressed. In that historic moment, both sexual "normality" and sex therapy were created. They've been related ever since.

It's good to know how most bodies typically behave. It's bad to think that's how your body must behave at all times and that, if it doesn't, there's something wrong with you. And it's destructive to think that your body has to behave a certain way in order for you to enjoy sex.

Imagining and creating the Sexual Response Cycle was an enormous accomplishment, and Masters and Johnson withstood career isolation, government surveillance, and death threats as their reward. That said, the model does contain some limits:

- It doesn't address desire, or how desire can affect the body's reactions.

- It implies that the same physical stimulation will always lead to the same outcomes.

- It doesn't address the reality that the same physical stimulation or activity can feel different at different times.

- It takes culture for granted rather than explicitly noting that the experiences of lab subjects—and the rest of us—are mediated by culture.

- Spirituality and other subjective experiences are not addressed.

- It assumes that orgasm is the normal conclusion of sexual events.

Since the model's development, various professionals have proposed revisions or other models of sexual functioning. Each addresses some of these criticisms. Still, the Masters and Johnson model is so much a part of our culture that people forget that it's just a model. It isn't an accurate description of everyone's experience. For example, as men get older, many don't climax with a partner—and they still enjoy sex. Similarly, some women climax through psychological stimulation alone. The Masters and Johnson model doesn't fit either of these cases.

Finally, it's important to remember that sex is rarely a continuous increase of desire, arousal, excitement, orgasm. For most people, arousal ebbs and flows during sex—whether because of external distraction, internal dialogues, the need to pee, their desire to talk, laugh, or rest, or the simple natural rhythms of their bodies. Viewing this natural ebb and flow as a problem or dysfunction is unrealistic and often a source of problems.

A Word About Orgasm

It's dessert, not the main course.

Okay, that's six words. But making orgasm the point of sex is a problem for two reasons:

- It makes it harder to have an orgasm.

- It devalues all sexual activities that don't lead to orgasm.

Orgasm generally lasts about, what—two, five, ten seconds? And sex, from the time you start taking off your clothes until the time you say, "That was nice" and reach for your BlackBerry, takes about, what—ten, twenty, thirty minutes? That means that orgasm is 1 percent or less of your total sex time. Making that 1 percent the point of the entire exercise seems rather foolish. And really not worth all the bother.

Some people find sex a little boring, and hope that a fabulous orgasm will somehow redeem the experience. That's like eating in a restaurant with uncomfortable chairs, bad service, and mediocre food—and hoping that dessert will be so great, it will make the whole frustrating experience worthwhile.

Well, they haven't invented a dessert that good, and they haven't invented an orgasm that good either. If sex makes you feel lonely, gives you a headache, confuses you about your partner's feelings, is physically painful, or is filled with avoidance and excuses, no orgasm in the world can make it all worthwhile.

Under these conditions, you might stop having orgasms too.

A better model? Do things you enjoy during sex. Get excited, please yourself and your partner. Include orgasm if you want to. But have sex that's so enjoyable that even if you don't climax, you'll feel it was time well spent.

How to Have a Baby—
Whether You Want to or Not

It's hard to relax, become intimate, and enjoy sex when we're concerned about creating a pregnancy unintentionally. And despite junior high school health class, many of us are still unsure about how babies are made—or prevented.

A woman needs three things to become pregnant: an egg, a sperm, and a place for them to hang out for nine months once they're hand-in-hand. All three have a limited shelf life.

Each month while a woman is fertile (roughly ages thirteen to fifty), one of her ovaries releases an egg ("ovulation"). That's when the window for the possibility of becoming pregnant opens wide. If that egg chances upon a fresh sperm, the pair could conceivably (!) implant somewhere (the "womb," the "Devil's incubator"), become a fetus, and ultimately, maybe, be born as a baby.

Here's the math: sperm can live for five days before an egg shows up. An egg can live for one or two days before a sperm comes along. So a woman can become pregnant for 2 + 5 days. Add a couple of days on each end for safety's sake, and that means that, *each month*, you and your partner are vulnerable for about eleven days. *You can become pregnant if you have unprotected intercourse during these eleven days.*

It's easy to know when a batch of fresh sperm is injected into the vagina. The question is: when is an egg available to team up with one of those sperm? Approximate answer: about halfway in between menstrual periods (that's what regulates the lining of the uterus, where a fertilized egg would implant and grow). In an average twenty-eight-day menstrual cycle, this corresponds to the second week and the beginning of the third week after the end of monthly menstruation. However, few cycles are exactly average, and any cycle can be thrown off by illness, stress, nursing, pheromones, abrupt changes in diet or sleep patterns, and other things.

If only you could predict exactly when you or your partner would ovulate, you'd have a great form of contraception—*if* you were absolutely, positively, rigidly unwilling to have intercourse during that open window of possible conception. A woman can estimate (but *only* estimate) when she'll ovulate by counting ten days from the beginning of her last period, but that's not terribly scientific. People who rely on this unscientific counting for birth control call it the "rhythm method." The technical term for these gamblers is "parents"; 25 percent of couples using this method become pregnant during a typical year. In the twenty-first century, taking this monthly risk is completely unnecessary and morally irresponsible.

Some people call this whole process the "miracle of life." Except it's no miracle—it's simple science. If you refuse to use real contraception, memorize and use these simple facts. Here's a chart that restates what I've just described:

How You Risk Creating a Pregnancy

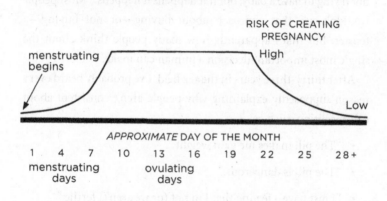

Contraception: Why Is It Special?
================================

For almost everyone, unintended pregnancy is *the* only serious thing that can go wrong with consensual sex.

Thus, effective contraception is a special part of Sexual Intelligence. When you've taken care of it, you can do whatever you like sexually; until you do, intercourse can have terrible consequences. That's no way to live, and no way to make love. When nothing can go wrong with intercourse, you can enjoy it in a very special way.

When intercourse can result in an unwanted pregnancy, how can a reasonable person relax and enjoy it?

To reduce both performance anxiety and normality anxiety, we have to make sex essentially harmless and meaningless. (If it's meaningless, you don't need to fear "failure.") This approach frees you to create profound, intimate, and personally meaningful sexual experiences; you and your partner just have to arrange your attitudes and behavior so that it doesn't really matter what happens during sex, as long as you both enjoy it.

I'm amazed at the casual approach many otherwise thoughtful people have about contraception.

When I ask patients about it, a surprising number say, "We're not trying to have a baby, but if it happens it happens." Most people wouldn't use that approach about buying—or not buying—a toaster. But that's apparently how many people think about the single most important decision a human can make.

After thirty-three years in the sex field, I've probably heard every reason supposedly explaining why people aren't consistent about contraception, such as:

- "The pill makes me gain weight."

- "The pill is dangerous."

- "I just have a feeling that I'm not (or we aren't) fertile."

- "Various methods interrupt spontaneity."

- "I'd feel pressured by all that planning."

- "I get (or she gets) no feelings with a condom."

- "I'm afraid I'll lose my erection putting on a condom."

- "We haven't been using birth control reliably for years, and nothing's happened yet."

- "A woman who plans to have sex is a slut."

- "I don't want any more kids, but what if I get sterilized and then my kids die in an accident? Or my spouse dies and my next spouse wants a kid?"

- "We don't agree on whether or not to have a kid (or another kid), and I don't want to fight every time we have sex."

- "I'm Christian and I'm not sure contraception is the right thing to do."

- "Maybe it's smart or well-off people like us who should be having kids."

- "I heard you can't get pregnant the first time (or standing up, or if you don't climax, or if the girl is on top, or if you shower afterwards, or if the guy pulls out)."

I do understand that discussing contraception can open up conversations you might not want to have—on topics such as:

- The future of the relationship

- The quality of your sex life

- Whether or not you're both sexually exclusive, and how you define that

- Conflict over whether or not you're going to have a child (or another child)

- Where you might be living in five years

- The unsettled question of whether one of you is ever going back to work

That's why contraception is more than just a technical activity; it can be the intersection of a number of emotional and relationship issues. When you haven't settled the principles and future of a relationship, avoiding birth control can be a way of avoiding other things. The problem is that the price for this avoidance can be an unintended pregnancy.

There's a contraceptive method for everyone, though each has its own inconveniences. Some people say, "I don't want any of the inconveniences associated with *any* of the methods, and therefore we'll use nothing." If people needed a license to have sex, that sort of thinking would be exactly what would disqualify someone. Expressing your sexuality in a safe, enjoyable, life-enhancing way is a glorious privilege. Making yourself vulnerable to a life-altering, unwanted consequence treats sex—and yourself—terribly disrespectfully.

Having intercourse? Fertile? Not 100 percent sure you want a pregnancy? To get more of what you want from sex, use contraception.*

Don't Forget the Morning-After Pill

Now here's an amazing invention: emergency contraception (EC). A carefully configured high dose of birth control pills, you can, depending on the brand, take it up to five days after unprotected intercourse, and it will prevent you from getting pregnant. *It's not an abortion pill* (that's a different drug, RU486), and it won't abort or affect a fertilized egg already implanted on the uterine wall. It just prevents pregnancy. Anyone who says differently is basing their opinion on something other than scientific fact.

Anyone seventeen or older can now get EC without a prescription. Its shelf life is several years. So if you're fertile and you don't

---

*For more information on contraceptive effectiveness and side effects, see web pages like "Women's Health" at http://womenshealth.about.com/cs/birthcontrol/a/effectivenessbc .htm, or "Comparing Effectiveness of Birth Control Methods" at http://www.plannedparenthood.org/health-topics/birth-control/birth-control-effectiveness-chart-22710.htm. When pursuing contraceptive supplies, advice, or information, make sure you're dealing with an organization that enthusiastically supports the availability and use of contraception. Not every organization purporting to give "advice" or "information" does that—and they're not always honest about it.

want to get pregnant right now, you should get some at your local pharmacy this week. Keep it around so that if your regular method fails (a condom breaks, your dog eats your birth control pills), you can protect yourself and your partner immediately. If you don't use it after three years, throw it away and buy a new package. Simply keep EC around as a matter of course, like toothpaste, balsamic vinegar, and AA batteries.

One year after you or your partner stops menstruating, you can stop buying EC. If you never used it, it was a good investment, a dollar a month for a very powerful kind of insurance. If you needed it, it was worth a million bucks. For more information on this modern wonder drug, see the Emergency Contraception website (http://ec.princeton.edu/questions/index.html).

Sexually Transmitted Infections

Then there's STIs. When I was growing up, it was called venereal disease. We thought "venereal" was Latin for "dirty, immoral, and shameful."

Many people consider an STI just about the end of the world. Once diagnosed they feel dirty, ashamed, broken. They wonder if anyone will ever again have sex with them, or if they'll ever be able to enjoy it again. They can't imagine ever telling someone about their condition.

Assuming you get treated, that's the worst set of consequences for every STI (except HIV) most people will encounter—shame, stigma, isolation. And some long-term relationships are damaged by the revelation (or suspicion) of infidelity that accompanies the diagnosis of an STI (which is why so many people keep the information from their partner).

Modern medicine makes it possible to deal with STIs the way we deal with other medical conditions. Bacterial infections like syphilis are cured with simple medication. Viral infections like herpes cannot be cured, but they can be managed with simple medication and lifestyle adjustments regarding diet and stress. In a small number of people, an untreated STI leads to infertility—but again, prompt treatment can prevent this.

In all, the lifelong consequences of an unintended pregnancy far, far outweigh the consequences of catching an STI.

Some people really care about STIs, and they use condoms or avoid genital/fluid sex. That's excellent; I want these folks to enjoy the sex they're having, not simply dread disaster. Many more people *say* they care about getting infected, but they don't do much to prevent it. Some of these people enjoy sex; some are too anxious to enjoy it.

Actually preventing the spread of STIs involves talking with your sexual partner(s). That can be unpleasant, but before you even get to that, let's note two things you can do that don't require any awkward conversation:

- Familiarize yourself with the outward symptoms of the most common STIs.*

- Casually check your partner for these symptoms, especially a new partner or one you haven't seen in a while. Showering together is an enjoyable way to do this. So is playing around with a partner's thighs, belly, and butt—in enough light that you can see what you're playing with.

But very, very few people do this. People really don't want to think about STIs. So why don't people "protect themselves"? And scientifically, what does "protection" mean?

- Limiting the number of your sexual partners

---

*See STI pictures at http://www.avert.org/std-pictures.htm (or Google "STI symptoms pictures").

- Periodically examining yourself (and knowing what you're looking for)

- Examining your partners (and knowing what you're looking for)

- Using nonfluid or nongenital forms of sex

- Using condoms for genital/fluid forms of sex

Very few people eagerly embrace all of these practices. The most that a lot of people can manage with a new partner is, "We should probably talk about, you know, disease. I don't have anything you need to know about. What about you? No? Great, let's proceed with abandon."

I know that many single and nonmonogamous men and women think about STIs, but generally the same way we Californians think about earthquakes—"I hope disaster doesn't strike, I know I should take precautions, but it's too much trouble, and if it happens, I'll just deal with it."

So why don't people deal with their anxiety or their rational concern about STIs?

- Who likes to acknowledge their partner's previous (sex) life?

- Who likes to acknowledge their partner's current (sex) life with others?

- Who wants to tell the truth about their previous or current sex life?

- Who wants to commit to condoms long-term?

By age fifty, one-quarter of the U.S. population tests positive for the genital herpes virus. Each year, over 1,000,000 people catch chlamydia, the country's most common STI. If you have one of these, or another STI, you are not alone. And you are neither dirty nor broken. But you will have to get treated, and you will have to learn how to talk about it.

Because people do die from diseases associated with HIV, we can't say that stigma and isolation are its worst consequences. But the risk factors for catching HIV are well known, and, statistically, most heterosexual Americans are not generally exposed to HIV. Nonmonogamous straight and gay people can protect themselves from HIV with reasonable decision-making regarding both sex and lifestyle choices.

Here's what I recommend:

- Consider the advantages of being really truthful with your sexual partner(s). The benefits go way beyond protection from STIs.

- Decide if your sex habits—present or past—put you at risk for HIV/AIDS. (This includes your partners' habits, right?) If so, get tested (it's private and free in most communities) this month, and think about whether or not you want to continue living this way.

- Get a routine blood test for common STIs. Inform your partner(s) of the results, even if they're negative (which could motivate them to get tested).

- Learn how to maximize pleasure during sex when you're using condoms (yes, there are tricks).*

- If you're fertile, get serious about birth control. It's *way* more important than STIs.

---

*For starters, use the right size; buy a few different brands, and compare. Make sure you and your partner are touching or kissing while the condom goes on. As it does, put a few drops of water-based (not oil-based) lube both inside the condom and outside (to promote the transfer of both heat and pressure—in other words, of sensation). Periodically, you or your partner should reach down and make sure the condom is snug at the base of the penis—a lovely opportunity to stroke the often-ignored scrotum ("balls," "nutsack"). For more tips, see an adult sex ed book or video.

Mars and Venus—Or Earth?

The last component of knowledge involves challenging the conventional wisdom about women and men.

Although we've all heard the expression "the opposite sex," I prefer "the other sex" or "the other gender." After all, men and women are not opposites. In fact, there's nothing on this earth that's more like a man than a woman. What's similar to a man— a fish, a pineapple, a rowboat, a sweater, an audiocassette, a glass of fresh lemonade? No. The thing on earth that's most like a man is a woman. And the thing on earth that's most like a woman is a man.

The idea that men and women communicate in vastly different ways may have a few tiny grains of truth to it, but the bigger picture is more important: sexually, men and women want the same things, are anxious about the same things, and withhold communication the same way. Both men and women are shy about bringing up herpes, shy about asking for a finger in their butt, and shy about saying, "Oh, do that harder," or "Please do that slower," or "Let's go brush our teeth first."

Let's remember there are over two billion adult women and over two billion adult men on this earth (and in late December it seems they're all at the mall at the same time). That makes today's "women" and "men" the biggest categories the world has ever seen. If you rely on those categories to understand your partner or yourself, you're going to miss a lot.

Are there any sure things you can rely on when making love with a man or a woman? Well, everybody needs oxygen to breathe, sooner or later everyone needs to pee, and everyone has a pain threshold. Of course, everyone's needs in all three departments vary widely.

Here are some other *almost*-sure things: most people want to feel special, most people want to feel attractive, and most people want to feel competent. So you can make assumptions in this direction, but pay attention in case your partner isn't one of these "most people."

And you? Get to know yourself; don't categorize yourself, and don't let your partner categorize you. When she says, "That's just like a man," tell the truth—"I do that because I'm me." If you don't stop for directions when you're lost, it isn't because you're a man, it's because you're foolish. And a woman who overspends at the shoe store isn't being just like a woman—she's being irresponsible.

The whole Mars/Venus idea that men and women are radically different creatures gets in the way of our relationships, making it hard to trust and enjoy them. How can people expect to relate meaningfully if they imagine they're from different planets?

Okay, so if men and women are so similar, why do so many people consider "the opposite sex" a problem? I think it's an understandable mistake of distance and focus. If you ask gay men who drives them crazy, they sigh and say, "Men." If you ask lesbians who drives them crazy, they frown and answer, "Women." That's because that's the gender of the people they're each sexual with. We already know who heterosexual people think is the problem—the other gender.

Most people have had negative dating experiences, and most of us occasionally get fed up with our significant other. We assign a range of negative characteristics to these characters we have loved, trusted, idealized, and been disappointed by: they're selfish, impulsive, bossy, passive, unreliable, manipulative, and they don't listen. And since most people are straight, this formulation sticks: men and women are "opposites" who keep betraying each other's dreams. But what people really mean, I think, is this: "Being in intimate relationships is hard! My partner is never perfect, and he (she) wants stuff!"

Here's a story that shows what happens when you base your marital and sexual decisions on "knowledge" that isn't factual—but you insist that it is. This is the opposite of Sexual Intelligence.

Both William and Hong grew up in Vietnam, and each still had parents living there. Without knowing each other, they had both come to San Francisco for college, and then stayed, pursuing separate lives. They eventually met, and although it wasn't exactly an arranged marriage, they each knew they were expected to marry a Vietnamese. And so even though Hong was divorced and eight years older than William, and even though they had very different personalities, they married a few months after being introduced.

That's when they started having sex. It was clumsy and frustrating, and after six months of trying, their enthusiasm began to wane. So after only two years of marriage, they came to see me.

William was intelligent, energetic, and likable, but his opinions were so rigid that they were hard to discuss, much less challenge. That was the marriage Hong found herself in. It didn't help the therapy to have William telling me, over and over, that he knew how things were for Vietnamese and I didn't. When Hong periodically complained that this was how he insulted her and everyone else, he would temporarily switch gears—dismissing what I'd say with a faux-gracious "everyone has their opinion, and we'll just have to agree to disagree."

It was aggravating, especially since they were clearly suffering, I liked them both, and I wanted to help them.

So what did William "know" about sex?

- Their chronic financial quarrels should not affect their desire or arousal.

- His low desire was at least partly because he was getting "older." ("I'm on the wrong side of thirty," he'd say.)

- It was wrong for an "older" woman to have as much sexual desire as Hong did.

- Marital sex should focus on intercourse, and Hong's
  request for "variety" (in her case, oral sex) wasn't part of
  "Vietnamese tradition." Therefore he didn't have to deal
  with these sexual interests.

Between sessions I'd make plans for how I would deal with
William next time. But despite my plans, each week I'd somehow
find myself debating him about the accuracy of his various assumptions. Sometimes I'd talk about narratives and constructed
reality, but that never went anywhere, since William was convinced
he was speaking truth, not simply giving his own perspective. So
I'd get pulled into discussions about the "normal" desire of forty-
five-year-old women, how common cunnilingus was in marriage,
how the human nervous system works, and so on. Week after week
I experienced exactly what Hong was up against.

Although Hong didn't really believe in the traditional model,
she was trying to be a good Vietnamese wife. But when she made
these attempts, her resentment would build, and his enormous
sense of entitlement (he wasn't just stubborn and narcissistic, he
was the firstborn son!) would become so hurtful and offensive to
her that she'd oscillate between withdrawal and sudden outbursts.
Then he'd be genuinely baffled: hurt that she had blown up at him,
and he'd actually expect an apology—which would infuriate her.

No wonder they didn't have sex.

I tried to explain to William that, at least here in the West, a good
sexual relationship was something two adults built collaboratively,
but he didn't hear it. Further, I urged him to speak to someone else
to get facts that would challenge his, but he refused. He said that
he respected me and that if he was going to reconsider his "facts,"
it would be with me. It was a flattering, but frustrating, moment.

Finally I suggested that Hong tell William she felt invisible to
him. He was sympathetic. I asked how that feeling compared to the
traditional mother and grandmother roles she had seen in Vietnam. "Just the same," she said bitterly. "As a girl, my grandmother

learned the rule of three obediences [to father, husband, and son].
Is that what my life is to be?" And her mother? "My father used to
threaten to divorce her if she didn't produce a son. And of course
she was a slave to my father's parents. Her reality was of very little
interest in that house."

   Asking William what sort of life he wanted, I said that I was very
sympathetic to his dilemma—should he have a traditional Vietnamese home or a more modern American one? In the former, his
word was law, and his "facts" were facts. In the second, his word
was more or less equal to his wife's, and his "facts" were subject to
challenge at any time. He thought about it for a long time. "I'm not
sure," he said slowly. "I want my marriage, but I don't like being
questioned, and I don't like the idea of being wrong."

   And if that made sex unenjoyable for her, or for him, or if it prevented satisfaction? "That might be necessary," he observed, "although it would be too bad." To his credit, William suggested that
they continue seeing me, but it was difficult to make progress with
him "knowing"—inaccurately—all that he did.

Both William and Hong were responsible for their sexual and marital problems. When people are in conflict, it's essential to separate fact from opinion, and opinion from ignorance or prejudice.
As the husband, William believed he had the privilege of not having to examine his "facts"—i.e., his assumptions, beliefs, and superstitions—about sex and gender. This, of course, made change
impossible.

Sexual Diversity

Stuck in his various stubborn positions (and claiming they weren't
stubborn positions), William didn't appreciate sexual diversity—

the wide range of how humans express their sexuality. His opinions about how others should live, and his beliefs about how others do live, were obstacles to a satisfying sex life and marriage.

So, unlike William, let's examine some actual facts about this diversity. These may help you relax during sex, and perhaps help you understand your partner or your experiences better.

- In sexuality, diversity among people is the rule, not the exception.

- In the human family, every dimension of sexuality is diverse—desires, fantasies, comfort level, risk-taking, orgasm, concepts of virginity, structures of sexual relationships, what's considered "kinky," and so on.

- For many people, the psychological context of their behavior is what makes sex exciting. This can include role-playing, enacting fantasies, wearing costumes, telling sexy stories, watching (or making) pornography, using code words, or being observed by others. For some people, a rough hand on the wrist, a simple black bra, or the words "Spank me, Daddy," or "Maybe we shouldn't do this," turn an ordinary event into a thrilling one. Other people find such things silly or unsexy.

- Millions of American adults are into "erotic power play"—consensual spanking, bondage, domination games, controlled humiliation, carefully calibrated intense stimulation, sensory deprivation, and so on.

- You can't tell what someone's sexual interests are based on the other things you know about him or her. For example, some people who are into rough sexual games come from rough backgrounds, while others come from mild and loving backgrounds. Some very ladylike and gentlemanly creatures get nasty and/or nutty between the sheets.

- "Men" and "women" are heterogeneous categories—they don't predict much about the sexuality of the people in

them. In fact, all categories are like that when it comes to
sex—of limited value.

I call this issue "diversity" rather than "normality" (see Chapter 2 on this) because my goal is not to allay your anxiety about
your normality. Rather, I want you to not *care* about whether your
sexuality is normal—to know that you can just be you. I want
to remind you about the wide range of what people do, some of
which probably makes no sense to you—just as some of what you
do would make no sense to people from other cultures or histori-
cal times.

For example, a Chinese patient of mine who came to the United
States for college thirteen years ago told me that the first time she
ever saw two adults kiss passionately was at the landing gate at the
Los Angeles airport. For a while she thought Americans were obsessed with not only kissing, but with kissing in public. A bunch of
osculo-exhibitionists!

Similarly, many people across the United States and around
the world keep some of their clothes on during sex. Others of us
wouldn't dream of doing so; in fact, we'd feel deprived of one of
our greatest pleasures during sex, skin-to-skin touch. Which way is
normal? Wrong question—because it doesn't matter. Do what you
and your partner find comfortable. (To expand your erotic vocabulary, see the hints throughout Part Three.)

This "diversity" issue is especially important if you're someone
who periodically tells your partner that she or he isn't normal, or
if you feel compelled to defend yourself from such an accusation.

Sexual Intelligence requires that you appreciate the concept of
sexual diversity. That doesn't mean you approve of every sexual
practice—although people around the world are not asking for
your approval to do what they do, thank you very much, any more
than you're asking for theirs.

Appreciating the concept of sexual diversity means that you

understand that *values*—subjective values—determine what a person, community, or culture considers sexually "normal," not some eternal truth. People and communities may claim that their values and judgments are inspired or dictated by "God," "common sense," or the "natural world," but it's all subjective, and all written by humans with human prejudices.

You can, of course, make the opposite, traditional argument, leaping to the defense of certain norms or alleged truths (it really doesn't matter which ones). But keep this in mind: if you tell your partner that his or her sexual preferences, fantasies, and limitations are not "normal" (instead of saying you're not comfortable with them), you're asking for trouble. Either your partner will agree, and shrink back from you accordingly, or disagree, in which case you'll have painful, irresolvable conflict. Claiming that you know what's "normal" is exactly the kind of power grab that undermines intimacy.

When you judge *yourself* according to some imagined standard of what's sexually normal, you're also asking for trouble. You're diminishing your individuality and comparing yourself to complete strangers. After all, you're not "people"—you're you. Thus, your sexuality doesn't need to resemble that of "other people."

Besides, a few centuries ago or a thousand miles away, you might be considered as normal as rain. Not that that matters, of course.

Chapter Five

Your Heart
Emotional Skills

Rowena came to see me because she was scared. She'd been caught having sex with a printer repair guy in her office right in the middle of the workday. Her boss told her that if she didn't fix her "sex addiction" immediately, she'd be terminated.

The twenty-six-year-old bookkeeper had only met the guy the previous day. She had this kind of semi-anonymous, semi-public sex periodically. And although she liked the danger of it (not to mention the orgasms), getting caught was a wake-up call. Was she just a good-time girl who loved sex, or was there something wrong with her?

She told me she was married, and that she loved her husband Jose. "But the adventure is gone," she said, shaking her head. "Maybe I shouldn't have gotten married. Do you think I'm just a sex addict?"

"I don't think 'sex addiction' is a helpful category," I told her. "I think some people have psychological problems—obsessive-compulsive disorder, bipolar disorder, borderline personality. But what others call 'sex addiction' I think is mostly people acting out sexually, and then not liking the consequences of their decision-making. Then these people say they're out of control—sexually 'addicted.'"

Rowena wasn't a "sex addict"; she struck me as someone who had unrealistic expectations about life and sex. So we talked about her need for adventure, the high of taking risks, the thrill of a new sex partner. Most importantly, we talked about how no matter how much she scratched she still had an itch, and the next casual encounter would be just around the corner. Maybe that was a clue, I said, that something else was going on.

"You mean, like when I masturbate two or three times during a day and I'm still horny?" "Exactly," I said. "Maybe you're using sex to get something that sex can't give you. And maybe that's preventing you from enjoying sex more deeply with your husband."

But as we continued talking, she got defensive. "Maybe you just think everyone should be married," she pouted. "Or that casual sex is just for guys. Maybe you're not the big sex-positive shrink everyone thinks you are."

"Actually, I don't care if you stay married or not," I said simply. "I'm more interested in you living with integrity, whatever that turns out to mean."

That was a surprise to her, and it got her thinking. After a minute's silence, she said, "You know, my reflexive feeling was, 'Well, I don't care if I stay married or not either.' How screwed up is that?"

This was a common pattern with us: she'd get angry with me or feel misunderstood, but eventually realize she'd been impulsive, and then emotionally re-enter our relationship.

Unconsciously, she used her sexuality with me that way also. While I'm certain she had no actual sexual intentions toward me, she did manage to tell me several times that she "loved giving head. I'm damn good at it too." Then she'd look at me and ask if she had embarrassed or upset me.

Rowena was trying to turn me into a controlling mother she could rebel against. This was, I soon learned, an eerie echo of her childhood, when she felt stifled by her strict Catholic mother. But Rowena had muted her adolescent resentment because her mother was sickly and physically weak. Rowena had to take care of her mother, which left little room to rebel—or to get much positive attention, either.

Enter a parade of Spanish tutors, UPS deliverymen, car mechanics, office repair guys, and even her dentist.

"You'll have to find ways of feeling important, loved, and pretty that don't involve casual sex if you want to enjoy being married," I said. "And I understand that might seem like an impossible task."

In fact it did. "But I can see that growing up is the only way out of this," she practically whispered. "How can I do that?"

Fast-forward through our first dozen sessions. It's been months of struggle. Rowena's been learning to stay more aware of her internal state, realizing what kind of emotional nourishment she needs at various times (exercise, hugs, laughter, meditation, self-validation, wholesome time with friends who care for her, and so on). And she's learning to talk more to her husband: more about being bored, more about wanting his self-disclosure, more about her reflex to rebel, even if she has to create an adversary to rebel against.

And they're talking more about sex. They've made a deal: she'll slow down and be more emotionally present during sex if he'll do the same.

"It's scary," she said. "I never thought sex could be scary until now. I guess that's progress, huh?"

* * *

Most grown-ups don't want to get into bed with someone if they're angry with or feeling hurt by them. So, for enjoyable sex, you need the skills to settle the non-sexual issues that come up during the week. You also need the skills to not get thrown by whatever happens during sex.

We all need emotional skills to create a relationship in which going to bed with someone makes sense. In case you haven't noticed, if you aren't dependable, cooperative, validating, appreciative, and caring—even when you're not especially in the mood—the times when you and your partner will both be up for sex won't come around too often.

We also need emotional skills to help us navigate the normal kinds of emotional events that can happen in bed—such as feeling lonely or abandoned, judged or criticized, self-critical, embarrassed, or ashamed, inadequate or disappointing to our partner. If you fall apart every time your partner doesn't orgasm, or every time you feel chubby, or every time you don't get exactly the emotional connection you want, sex will become less and less enjoyable—and eventually less and less frequent.

And I haven't even mentioned the more specific things that happen during sex—like getting a cramp in your foot, wetting the bed, needing to stop in the middle, or climaxing unexpectedly. Do you have the emotional skills to handle situations like these? Over time that's definitely more important than dependable erections or lubrication on demand.

Events like these are about emotions—not about "sex" or our genitalia. As with every other activity (going to parties, watching movies, sitting on the beach, listening to music), during sex our body does what it does; we then assign meaning to what it does (or doesn't do), and *that's* what can create trouble. These emotional events also involve interpreting your partner's behavior, whether it's lack of orgasm, or the look on your partner's face when you undress, or your partner's refusal to touch you in a certain way or to accept how you want to touch him or her.

The same skill that helps you handle yourself when your partner forgets your birthday or wants to go to the ballet the day of the Super Bowl also allows you to handle not getting oral sex when you hope for it, or being told that your partner doesn't want to share pornography with you.

Most sex therapists say that a lot of their work isn't about sex itself. Rather, they're often helping people develop relationship skills and personal maturity, which ultimately make cooperation much easier. But this takes time, and not everybody wants to do it.

I was unable to do this effectively with Zena and Lamar.

Zena's distress about Lamar's lack of sex drive had brought them into my office. Maybe "distress" gives the wrong idea. She was angry, blaming, sarcastic, and sometimes just unapologetically nasty. Believe it or not, none of these made him more interested in sex with her.

She had plenty of reasons to be disappointed. He was what most people would call a slob—dropping his socks and underwear anywhere he happened to undress. He never capped or closed anything—toothpaste, peanut butter, dresser drawers. Not only did he scratch wherever it itched, he farted and belched at will, laughing when she complained.

"You're immature," she would complain session after session. "You're controlling," he would reply. "Hostile," she'd announce. "No sense of humor," he'd respond. After six weeks of this, I started hoping they would call and cancel their next session, or maybe quit therapy altogether.

While Lamar was no picnic, Zena was the tougher one to work with. Whenever I tried to process their mutual hostility, she'd turn on me. And when I noted that her goal of making him feel bad ("so he'll change") was creating problems of its own, she blew up at me. After a few of these ugly incidents, I noticed I was starting to withdraw from her. Of course, that's what Lamar was doing too, which drove her crazy. So one week I stepped up and talked about how I was becoming hesitant to engage Zena—that is, to tell her the truth—just as I imagined Lamar had become hesitant. I thought that describing my own dynamic with them might provide new insight that they could use. Alas, she blasted me with a "you men are jerks" speech, completely erasing my individuality as she lumped me into a category with her husband and two billion other jerks.

No, I did not like this. But I sure was experiencing what it was like to be in a relationship with her.

I learned that it was more effective to explain things to Lamar than to Zena; not only would she get less defensive, but she liked the idea that I was "working on him, the one with the problem."

Despite this, whenever I came too close to the subject of how she was treating him, she'd get terribly upset and defensive. Finally, I had to just say it: when people don't get along outside the bedroom, they often have trouble getting into the bedroom—much less enjoying what goes on there. He nodded. She exploded. Apparently, she wanted to be right more than she wanted to be sexually engaged with him.

For one thing, she wanted it clear that she was *not* to blame for their problems, and she wanted it clear that she was disappointed with her selection of a husband, who was apparently quite defective. When I suggested that having a sex life might require her to accept some responsibility for how things had unraveled, she became mean. So I gently suggested she might be feeling attacked by what I'd just said. This was apparently her cue to get sarcastic. So I backed off, and it took another month before I could even approach the subject again.

Zena and Lamar eventually left counseling without settling their sexual issue. And she did it in a predictably hostile way: she left me a voice mail saying they'd just had another fight, that the counseling was a waste of time, and that she had told him he needed individual therapy or she'd leave him. And that I shouldn't expect a call from either of them, because he agreed with her.

Zena refused to even consider acquiring new emotional skills in order to improve her sexual relationship. So what emotional skills go into Sexual Intelligence?

Self-Acceptance

"The first thing I learned about sex was shame."

This is what a patient told me during my first month as a therapist. I never forgot it.

When we don't accept ourselves, it's almost impossible to imagine someone else accepting us. Think about it—if you don't like your own cooking, can you imagine someone else enjoying it? If you think you're a boring person, do you believe someone who says you're fascinating?

It's the same with sex. We need to accept ourselves—our bodies, our preferences, our experiences, the way we orgasm (or don't)—in order to imagine that our partner accepts or even celebrates us. Without self-acceptance, we're constantly on the defensive. Someone says you look great? You respond with an apology, defensiveness, or suspicion that you're being patronized.

If you can't accept yourself, how can you approach your partner to create—much less enjoy—a sexual space between the two of you? If, for example, you have a neurotic fear of somehow hurting your partner with your masculinity, you'll withdraw and limit emotional contact with her. She'll undoubtedly experience this as hurtful—which was exactly what you wanted to prevent. At that point you can forget about having relaxed, playful sex—perhaps any sex at all.

Self-acceptance is a key resource in unhooking from sex that's oriented toward "normality" and performance. It allows you to put your own experience in the center of your sexual decision-making, rather than feeling trapped by conventional societal ideas that may not suit you. It's self-acceptance that enables you to tell a partner you'd rather do X (your thing) than Y (everyone else's supposed thing), which is crucial to enjoyable sex.

Similarly, self-acceptance can give you the confidence and relaxation to allow a partner to be himself or herself. When both of you are willing to be yourselves, you're on the way to sex you can both enjoy.

So "improving yourself" is *not* the centerpiece of making sex better. Start by accepting yourself the way you are—big butt, small penis, unpredictable orgasm, whatever—without "improvements."

I fondly recall a patient named Christopher, who came to therapy because his wife complained he was passive in bed. She insisted that he was passive because he didn't find her exciting, but that was absolutely wrong. Christopher just didn't feel entitled to get really excited, to make requests (much less demands), to ever pull her toward him the way she yearned to be.

Christopher grew up in a small Oklahoma town where his family owned the only grocery store. His parents worked constantly to keep the store open almost around the clock, and they expected Christopher and his brothers to pitch in every day. The message of his childhood was simple: life is hard, don't complain, work is everything, survival is the goal. And if you have any feelings or needs, keep them to yourself.

At seventeen, Christopher escaped to a Jesuit seminary in Oregon. Although he appreciated the intellectual stimulation, the place simply reinforced his family's message about the centrality of sacrifice, adding a crucial twist—sex is not a legitimate need. By the time he finally left the seminary ten years later (and became, of all things, a nurse), he had relationships all figured out: never focus on your needs, don't do anything that might be considered selfish, and do not exploit others with your desires.

Facing an adult world without having accepted his own needs and interests, Christopher found it impossible to really hunger after his wife. And he found it equally impossible to talk about his distress about this. Our therapy started with a goal that seemed simple, but was totally profound: knowing what he wanted, admitting it to himself, and then sharing it with her. That was way more important than teaching him a new position or getting her to wear lingerie.

Trust

I see a lot of men and women who tell me they have "trust issues." I tell them, "Ah, so you're uncomfortable trusting." I like that formulation better—it's easier to change a "discomfort" than an "issue." "Trust issues" sounds soooooo serious—who could be optimistic about changing that? Besides, "trust issues" sounds like the problem is external, like being hit by a bus, or having airport security mistake you for a terrorist. "I feel uncomfortable trusting" pulls the problem down to a human scale that can actually be changed.

There are many things you need to trust during sex: that pleasure is safe and appropriate; that eroticism won't get out of control in a destructive way; that you can connect with someone without being exploited; that your partner is telling the truth when he or she expresses desire, arousal, or satisfaction with you.

But you also need to trust *yourself*. Too many people are told all their lives that doing so is a mistake. My patient Douglas, for example, has never trusted himself. With parents who told him he was no good, who compared him (unfavorably) with cousins, neighbors, and everyone else, he grew up with no sense of entitlement. He feared speaking up or wanting anything because he believed that humiliation was sure to follow.

How could a person like this connect with someone sexually? He would be concerned about his erections, about coming too soon, about not being a good kisser. But these technical matters would be the least of his problems. Without trusting himself, he wouldn't trust sex or his partner. Being betrayed by his genitalia would be only the start of his problems; his anxiety and self-criticism would be the central feature of sex for him. Think he could enjoy it? No.

It turns out that trusting ourselves is fully as important as trusting others.

Communication

Most people don't realize that when couples have problems, communication is typically an *emotional* skill, not a *technical* one.

No matter how clearly and responsibly you intend to express yourself, it's hard to communicate well when you fear conflict or abandonment, have trouble trusting, or can't accept that neither you nor your partner is perfect. That's when communication is no longer about techniques and listening—it's about the emotions that prevent us from using those techniques and prevent us from listening. To improve communication at that point, we have to deal first with those emotions.

Communication is like many other activities, such as driving, cooking, and public speaking. If you're comfortable doing them, if you think people like you can be good at them, if you're not terrified of making a mistake, then you can enjoy such activities and become skillful at them, even creative. At that point these are merely technical skills.

But if you're *not* comfortable being a person who drives or cooks or speaks in public without worrying about being watched and judged, then your emotional difficulty is far more important than your technical skills. You can't learn or do these activities easily—not because you're stupid or clumsy, but because you're afraid or uncomfortable.

And so one of this book's goals is to turn communication from an emotional issue into simply a technical one.

I have so many patients who are told—by magazines, the Internet, various TV personalities—to communicate more or differently. Their partners often tell them in meticulous detail what they're doing wrong, wanting them to change. My patients generally feel that this trivializes their difficulties; frustrated and discouraged, they then say things like, "I just want to kiss you, but all I get is criticism," or, "Can't we do one single thing without wasting a lot of time communicating?"

While some people do refuse to communicate ("it's none of your business," "you don't really care," "you just want to control me, like my ex"), most don't. Rather, people who are verbally restrained or who hide behind euphemisms are typically just so bound up that communication is almost impossible. For them communication is an emotional skill, rather than a simply technical one.

That's why they often answer questions with just one syllable, or they "forget" to start conversations. They're scared or intimidated, not mean or stingy.

Take Manush, for example, an almost reclusive lab technician who was finally dating again many years after his lover died. He thought the main goal of communication was to prevent his current boyfriend, Carl, from getting upset. Manush tiptoed around him; in fact, he often waited until they'd both had one or two drinks at night before talking about difficult things.

Out of practice, concerned about losing Carl, Manush was looking for the "right way" to communicate—instead of relaxing and drawing on their connection. He still couldn't accept that Carl wouldn't always be happy with what he said or wanted. He hesitated to have the more adventurous sex that Carl wanted because he didn't want to get that wrong either.

After two months of therapy, in which we talked about his fears of communicating, he started "coming out" to Carl: An "I'd like" here. A "maybe we could" there. A mild challenge now and then to Carl's assumption of being in charge. Confronting Carl's belief that he knew Manush better than he knew himself. He was scared at first, but the more Manush did it, the more he realized how important it was to do—and how not doing so all along had actually undermined, not strengthened, the relationship.

At that point it made sense to talk about the technicalities of communication—"I" statements (talking about your experience rather than your partner's supposed intentions), fair fighting (staying on topic, not bringing up old hurts), striving to understand before striving to be understood (the opposite of what most people in conflict do). And that's when things really got interesting. The occasional conflict meant they had sex less often—but finally, the sex between them could heat up. They both loved it. Much to Carl's delight, they started to experiment with sex toys and games that Manush had thought were only for other people. How pleased he was to be wrong about that!

Regardless of the topic, the goal of communication isn't to satisfy your partner or to get your partner off your back; it's to be more present and to have more power to shape your relationship experiences.

Growing Up

I wish I could say, "C'mon, just grow up," to some of my patients who are trying hard to succeed in our therapy—but of course this doesn't help (I tried it as a rookie shrink), and it isn't good therapy.

When was the last time you said, "C'mon, just grow up" to someone and they actually did?

Still, there's no substitute for growing up if you want a better relationship or want to enjoy sex more. That's because of the common tendency to use sex as a substitute for grappling with the fears and anxieties of adulthood.

When you've worked out those fears—of being unattractive, for example, or irrelevant, or not sufficiently manly—it's easier to have sex that's just about sex. In contrast, when sex is about concerns like whether or not you're still youthful, or lovable, or important, sex—along with your genitalia—is just carrying too much of a burden. Expecting your penis to determine whether or not you're still relevant, or expecting orgasm to distract you from your fear of dying, is just putting too much pressure on small pieces of flesh. No wonder penises and vulvas sometimes refuse to cooperate.

Part of dealing with these existential issues is coming to peace with your body as it is. This involves letting your body be what it is during sex and imagining that your partner accepts it too. There's nothing so offputting as telling one's partner, "I like your body" (or this body part), only to be contradicted: it's too fat, too skinny, too wrinkled, the wrong shape or color. No one wants their opinion invalidated, certainly not their positive opinion of their partner's body. In addition, wrangling over the attractiveness of a body or body part creates distance—generally the opposite state that people have in mind when they're appreciating their partner's body.

Being grown-up also involves accepting that tragedies are part of life. When you do, it becomes easier to put a lost erection in perspective—it is *not* a tragedy. In fact, if you learn to laugh at what life throws at you, it's easier to laugh at the vagaries of sex, which makes it easier for you and your partner to relax.

I recall one patient who couldn't grow up enough to forgive her husband for being himself—a nice guy who would never make a fortune. Whenever Elise became anxious about money or felt envious of well-to-do people, she would make snide remarks about how she'd be living in a much nicer house if only she had married her first boyfriend (who became a corporate lawyer) instead of Eduardo (who was a carpenter).

Periodically distraught about her life choices, Elise simply couldn't maintain sexual desire for Eduardo. She acknowledged that he was attractive and a gentle, patient lover—but the grief she felt when she looked at him simply prevented her from appreciating or desiring him. Unfortunately, therapy couldn't help her come to terms with the life she had chosen for herself—and for her own reasons, she was unwilling to change her choice.

Maintaining Sexual Self-Esteem in the Face of Disappointment

If you know you're smart, your intelligence isn't on the line every time you go to work. If you know you're a good mother, your confidence as a parent isn't on the line every time you manage a disagreement with your kids.

Wouldn't it be nice if you could decide that you're sexually competent and attractive (at least to your mate)? That way, your sexual adequacy and self-esteem wouldn't be on the line every time you have sex. The ways your body responds during sex wouldn't "mean" anything; although you might feel disappointed if you didn't get what you hoped for, your attitude about yourself wouldn't change.

If your opinion of yourself varies with the outcome of each sexual encounter, you'll continually be pressuring yourself to do sex "right" (erection, lubrication, orgasm, timing, whatever)—and that makes enjoyment very difficult. It makes each sexual encounter too meaningful—as if *this* is the time you find out if you're loved, or attractive, or adequate. And that makes every sexual encounter an opportunity to fail. Who can enjoy that?

While it's enjoyable to feel that sex has *personal* meaning, it's best when the outcome of a sexual encounter determines nothing. Disappointment is *not* the same thing as failure. Disappointment is a reasonable response to the difference between what you want and what you get. Failure is a global judgment about who you are, as demonstrated by the difference between what you want and what you get.

An example? The millions of women who insist that when a man doesn't get erect, or ejaculates too quickly, *she* is a failure. This expectation puts pressure on both partners, who may eventually start avoiding sex in order to avoid embarrassment and loss of self-esteem.

Tolerating Inadequate Attunement

"Attunement" is how I describe the experience of two (or more) people inhabiting a common psychological space at the same time. People refer to this variously as "being on the same page," "thinking with one brain," "taking the words right out of my mouth," "reading my mind," or "being in synch."

More practically, people say things such as, "When we cook together, it's like we're dancing in the kitchen." "On a good day, we can get all three kids up, dressed, fed, and out the door without saying a word to each other." "Right before hosting a big party, we're like a well-oiled machine getting everything done together."

Whether through coparenting, playing doubles tennis, hosting dinner parties, attending the Super Bowl, or playing in a string quartet, many people yearn for the feeling of attunement—the sense of joining others in a common experience. It can be a wonderful human pleasure.

Another way people like to do this is through sex, which they may describe as "being touched the way I've always wanted to be touched," "our bodies talking to each other perfectly," or "making love like we've known each other forever."

But it doesn't always unfold that way, does it? In fact, for some people, sex *never* feels like this—from the moment they start kissing or someone starts undressing them, it's all elbows and knees. And they feel so grief-stricken or enraged about it that they can't enjoy anything else sex has to offer.

For other people, sex works fine until it doesn't—and then it *really* doesn't. Like their cousins just described, they suddenly feel hurt or lonely or abandoned, to a degree way beyond what a specific situation seems to merit (a lost erection, an accidental hair pull, a disagreement about who's going to get on top, feeling tickled instead of caressed).

When that happens, sex is the least of their problems. Depending on their character style, they may lash out or emotionally collapse. Suddenly there's a relationship problem (or "drama," as their partner may complain); some couples, in fact, always seem to be stumbling from one of these conflicts to the next.

It's hard to be enthusiastic about sex when you don't know how to tolerate the disappointment of insufficient attunement. Eventually, such people hesitate to initiate or respond sexually. Their partner loses enthusiasm too. Since no one gets that sense of attunement from sex (or from anything else) every single time, Sexual Intelligence gives you the ability to tolerate *not* having it when you want or expect it.

While the desire for attunement during sex can be perfectly healthy, some adults put way too much emphasis on it. Perhaps they unconsciously yearn to experience the profound attunement they didn't get enough of as a child. Particularly if they feel they deserve such attunement, or if sex is laden with mystical meaning for them, the lack of attunement during sex can be excruciating.

Unfortunately, their partner may make things worse by criticizing such an intense response to a provocation that may seem minor. The upset person then feels the additional pain of their partner apparently trivializing their distress.

Predictably, people who can't tolerate a lack of attunement soon reveal this in therapy. Every week I deal with patients attempting, consciously or not, to manipulate, whine, bully, or seduce their way into a sense of attunement with me. Their fondest wish is that I will acquiesce to this "invitation." Instead, I generally comment on their desire—which often leads them into a terribly familiar sense of disappointment right in session. That's when serious personal growth is possible—for those who have the patience and determination to examine their feelings rather than insist that I and others have done something wrong. Not everyone does, of course. You can see how this kind of self-observation contributes to Sexual Intelligence—the ability to enjoy sex when the situation isn't perfect.

I recall working with a woman named Malika who'd grown up in a privileged home in Karachi, Pakistan. There, the servants were trained to not just *satisfy* her, but to *anticipate* her material and emotional needs. Raised to expect this treatment, she never learned how to cope with everyday frustration while growing up. This wouldn't have been such a problem if she'd stayed in Pakistan, either living in her father's house or marrying a rich man. But she did neither—she went to California for college, and stayed there afterwards. She then married an American—a nice enough engineer, but a middle-class guy who was clueless about what he was getting into.

Four years later, she came for therapy, assuring me that the problem was her "unsophisticated" husband, who was driving her crazy with "suburban ideas." She couldn't feel desire for such a "pedestrian fellow," someone who "didn't have stars in his eyes."

The first few times Malika felt frustrated with me in therapy she was quite vocal and snooty about it. Working with her to build a respectful adult relationship with me was a big—and slow—step toward building her tolerance for disappointment, especially where her husband was concerned. She had to learn to appreciate the small satisfactions in everyday life, and to accept that not every moment in her life would be filled with "stars." She wanted children, for example, but was planning on them being gifted, self-disciplined, perfectly behaved, and tidy—virtually effortless to raise, of course. Was she in for a surprise!

How does this connect with sex? When Malika learned she could survive imperfect moments—a tired husband, a bruised banana, a rude waitress, a doctor keeping her waiting—down-to-earth sex became easier. Until our work together, she had experienced love-making as a series of assaults on her five senses—such as not being touched perfectly, the room not being the perfect temperature, her husband not being perfectly shaved. As our therapy proceeded, she stopped constantly criticizing her poor husband and started to notice what she *was* enjoying about sex.

I knew we were making progress the day a car alarm went off in the parking lot below my office window and she was able to continue the session. Thanking me for my insights (and patience!), she said, "I suppose if I can talk with you while that's happening, I can even make love with my husband when the world isn't perfect."

Now *that's* using your Sexual Intelligence.

And So . . .

Emotional skills are like oxygen—invisible, and unnoticed unless missing. We talk about emotional skills primarily when they're lacking. But the emotional skills of adulthood are essential for desiring and creating enjoyable sex. These skills enable us to relate to sexual situations that aren't ideal, which may be the majority of our experiences. And they enable us to deal with a partner who inevitably must struggle with imperfect sexual experiences too.

Perfect bodies? Perfect "function"? They're worth very little in the real world of adult sexual expression. Maturity, patience, perspective, a sense of humor? Now *that's* sexy.

Chapter Six

Your Body
Awareness and Comfort

You may recognize the following dynamic, which is common among many couples. I hear about this pattern so often that I'll give it to you in a basic, stripped-down version.

Once again, Max unintentionally leans on Trina's hair, or squeezes her nipple too hard, bangs her pubic bone, pushes his tongue too far into her mouth, or rubs her clitoris too roughly.

> Frustrated (and perhaps temporarily in pain), Trina criticizes Max for being a selfish oaf.

> Max tries harder (this time or next time) to do what Trina wants, which makes him feel anxious, which makes it even harder to make fine motor adjustments in his touch. As a result, Max's behavior doesn't change enough for Trina to notice.

> Getting more frustrated, Trina feels emotionally distant and more critical.

> Max feels more anxious and inept; he feels ashamed about being unable to please his partner.

Trina gets more frustrated and doesn't give as many helpful cues.

Feeling overwhelmed by her distancing, Max pulls back.

Trina feels abandoned and uncared for.

Hurt and confused, Trina eventually decides that Max's inability to be physically attuned with her is his "fault" and that it reflects his lack of commitment to her. He attempts to "try harder," which rarely works. But he knows he cares for her, that he wants to please her, and that he's trying hard. Her interpretation—that he's uncaring—hurts him very much. He ultimately decides that she's overly sensitive and impossible to satisfy.

They don't discuss their mutual sadness much, eventually deciding that they "have a sex problem."

Now they're really in trouble.

✳ ✳ ✳

Sexuality involves bodies, each belonging to a separate person. In the last chapter, we talked about how sexual partners typically enjoy having their bodies attuned to each other, and feel disappointed when they aren't. Sexual Intelligence informs us that, for most people, this attunement is essential in order for sex to feel "intimate."

In this chapter, we look at the nuts and bolts of this attunement, both how to maximize it and what can interfere with it.

Three-Dimensional Radar and Our Sixth Sense

For bodies to be attuned to each other, two things must be involved:

a. You know *how to control* your body's movements (proprioception).

b. You sense *how your body relates* to its environment— which includes another body (kinesthetic awareness).*

These skills involve the internal ability to sense your own body. Even blindfolded, you know if your arm is above your head or hanging by your side; with your eyes closed, you can probably touch your finger to your nose. Try it; it's actually pretty amazing. Sexual Intelligence requires both of these skills, so you can relate your body to your partner's body without much thought or effort. It's not about sexual "function" or "dysfunction"; it's about the ability of two bodies to find and relate to each other.

Proprioception is the sensory input and feedback mechanism that tells the brain about body position and movement without requiring conscious thought. Its receptors are located within muscles, joints, and connective tissues, as well as in sense organs and the inner ear. Your brain receives feedback about your body every second. It processes this information routinely so it can command your body parts to move smoothly, keep you balanced, and modulate your voice. You know the five senses? Proprioception is a sixth sense, your "position sense."

Kinesthetic awareness is the ongoing, always-changing sense of where your body is in time and space. It isn't enough to control

---

*Of course, you also need the emotional skills to *tolerate being that close* to another person and their body. We discussed some of these skills in the previous chapter, and will continue later in this chapter.

your body's movements—you have to make the right movements to accomplish what you want. Do you want to get close to someone's face, or accidentally lean on their hair? Do you want to smell someone's chest, or accidentally bang your nose into it? Kinesthetic awareness is your body's three-dimensional radar—again, without constant conscious awareness.

An activity like skiing requires both skills working together: proprioception gives you the reflexive sense of what your limbs must do to keep you upright. Kinesthetic awareness lets you know where your body is in relation to the skis and the slope so you can adjust your angle, speed, and direction.

Another example is everyday speech. It's one (physical) skill to know how to create a certain volume; it's a separate (physical) skill to know how your voice at a given volume sounds; a third skill—cognitive, not physical—decides if your voice is the correct volume for the situation; then we're back to the first skill of adjusting the volume so it's the level you're aiming for. When you're in a romantic little cafe and the idiot at the next table is yelling into his cell phone, you don't know if he realizes how loudly he's talking, or just doesn't care, or perhaps even thinks it's appropriate. Each of those involves a different skill (for the idiot).

How does this relate to sex? Here's an example: Proprioception gives you the sense of how to move your arms to hug someone. Kinesthetic awareness lets you know how far you need to reach, and what the strength of your hug needs to be so that the recipient gets the hug you intend. Then of course there's the social skill of judging whether or not this person wants a hug from you—yet a third part of the situation.

When Instincts Don't Quite Work

Athletic trainers, ballerinas, and child development experts find this topic endlessly fascinating. But most of us just take these two unconscious skills for granted—until there's a problem. In fact, deficits in these two skills create a lot of disruption in sexual relationships. But most people don't think about these instincts, so they don't realize that difficulties with one or both could be the source of a problem.

For example, when people have proprioceptive difficulty, they have trouble with:

- Instinctively knowing what various parts of the body need to do in order to move a certain way
- Instinctively knowing how much pressure is needed to, say, stroke an arm or squeeze a breast

Similarly, when people have difficulty with kinesthetic awareness, they have trouble:

- Accurately estimating what their body's movements feel like to someone else
- Accurately estimating how close they are to another person, the speed at which they're actually moving toward or away from that person, and the extent to which two movements are similar or different

We might describe problems like these as neuro-sexual learning disabilities. Note that this is completely different from someone saying, "Please don't touch me that way," and the other person saying, "Aw, c'mon, there's nothing wrong with me touching you that way. Get over it." And of course people frustrated with these problems don't typically imagine that they have such a disability.

To their partner, people with these disabilities appear clumsy or self-absorbed or uncaring. Their partners may get impatient or resentful, assuming that if the other person would just pay more attention and be more caring, they wouldn't keep leaning on them the wrong way, accidentally pulling their hair, or "whispering" too loudly in their ear.

But just as some people's eyesight or hearing isn't great no matter how much they "pay attention," so it is with proprioception and kinesthetic awareness.

Here's a simple way to check yourself or a partner. We know that someone who is always asking others to speak louder often has a hearing problem; that's also true if a person is always complaining that their partner speaks too loudly. If your partner says "ouch" a lot in bed, or sex keeps getting interrupted by complaints of being kicked, elbowed, or bitten too hard, one of these neuro-sexual difficulties may be responsible. If so, both you and your partner need to think about the situation as a physical problem rather than a character flaw—and approach it as a learning disability.

Of course, some people really are self-centered or uncaring. But those who genuinely struggle with a lack of instinct about their own body—whether they realize they're struggling or not—should be able to explore it in a cooperative environment. People have to talk about how to handle this deficit, just as they would with a partner who has a poor memory or suffers from ADD.

On the one hand, a sexual partner with a high degree of proprioception generally will seem technically proficient. And a sexual partner with a high degree of kinesthetic awareness will seem empathic and sensitive. The ideal lover, of course, has plenty of both skills (and great hair and plenty of money, but that's another story).

When making love with someone who has poor proprioception, however, you might think, *He's very clumsy,* or, *She doesn't know what to do in bed.* When making love with someone who has reasonable proprioception but lacks kinesthetic awareness, you might get the impression that *he's a great athlete, but he doesn't connect with me,* or *she's great in bed, but there's just something missing,* or *he's gorgeous, but he's too involved with himself.* In general, we criticize sexual partners who lack one or the other of these instinctive abilities, thinking their behavior reflects unacceptable emotional or character traits—uncaring, selfish, bossy, aggressive, bitchy, crude.

The worst combination, of course, is when an undersensitive person ("A") gets together with an oversensitive person ("B"). That's when it seems like A has two settings for touch—too hard and too soft—while B needs for A to have two hundred settings in between those extremes, and wants to be touched at exactly one (and only one) of those two hundred settings. Similarly, one person may be able to distinguish only the color red, while his or her partner can see dozens of shades of red, orange, pink, and gold. Now imagine this couple being clothes designers or offset printers, occupations in which color distinctions are critical.

Unfortunately, the way the brain processes and responds to the body's internal feedback can be disrupted by trauma or bad experiences, past or present. In fact, anxiety itself (including anxiety about being "clumsy") can disrupt your internal feedback process—including the common self-pressure in sex of trying desperately to do certain things.*

This sounds like a ballplayer pressuring himself so much that he has trouble catching a ball, doesn't it? In contrast, when we say that an athlete performs well under pressure, we mean that he can handle that external pressure without disrupting his processing, feedback, and motor functioning. In other words, he doesn't respond to *external* pressure by creating damaging *internal* pressure.

---

*There are ways to improve your proprioception and kinesthetic awareness. The first step is getting assessed by a neurologist, physiatrist, or sports medicine specialist. Modalities such as Feldenkreis, Pilates, and Alexander Technique can be helpful in increasing your body awareness and learning to self-monitor, along with yoga, tai chi, juggling, and working with a trainer on a wobble board, balance balls, and other gym equipment.

Some people consciously use tricks to do this (such as visualization or memory cues). Others are more natural at it.

Touching Can Be Complicated

There's another physical aspect of sexuality: the affinity for *touching*. Some people just don't like to be touched that much, while others love it. We shouldn't be surprised about this—after all, it's unusual when two people have the same level of interest in anything, whether it's sunsets or mac-and-cheese or Gwyneth Paltrow films.

As with everything else, each of us starts life with our own unique level of interest in touching. But how we respond to touching is more than just a matter of personal taste; some babies are apparently more sensitive to stimulation than others. They hear, smell, feel, taste, and see things more intensely, which can be terribly disconcerting. Such babies quickly get a reputation for being picky about the way they're fed or held, and they don't handle changes in the environment (a light turned on, a noise outside, dad's post-workout smell) that well.

Understandably, they don't gratify their caretakers with lots of smiles and cooing, which is the worst baby sin of all.

These extra-sensitive babies attempt to communicate at least as much as other babies, through vocalizations and gestures, like motioning to be picked up or pointing at a desired toy. But they're typically less successful than other babies because they're in more distress, have more specific demands, and do fewer attractive things. Their ultimate desire—"less intense stimulation, please!"—is of course impossible for them to convey, difficult for parents to conceptualize, and hard for anyone to accommodate.

Now fast-forward thirty years.

Some adults who are overly sensitive to stimulation may express it by a distaste for touch, body smells, the moisture of sex, and so on. They can appear to be anti-sex, just as they may also appear to be anti-music, anti-food, anti-clothes, anti-shopping, and anti–other people's laughter. But that may not be true; it may simply be that the normal intensity of sex, like these other things, is too overwhelming for them to handle comfortably.

Such discomfort can be baffling if you're someone who craves touch, enjoys sexual intimacy and pleasure, and feels deprived by your partner's physically reserved nature. And if you're convinced that your partner's quirkiness is about you—if you're taking his or her distaste for touch or sex personally—that can make productive conversation about this almost impossible. Sexual Intelligence reminds us not to take our partner's preferences, limitations, or "function" personally. It's one of the most important ways to keep sex free of performance anxiety.*

The Emotional Side of Body Issues

Having looked at our physical equipment and its vagaries, let's look at some of the ways you need to be emotionally comfortable with your body regarding sex. Because even with the most finely developed physical instincts, you need to cope with a wide range of issues just to enjoy a simple sexual encounter.

Sexual Intelligence recognizes this reality, and it provides tools for getting comfortable with the messiness of sex—both literally and figuratively.

---

*Many clinical professions offer successful ways of enhancing comfort with, and interest in, touch: physical and occupational therapists; yoga, dance, and massage instructors; psychologists; sex therapy with a surrogate partner; and hypnotherapists who do guided visualizations. Couples can participate in most of these modalities together.

Sex Is Messy—Literally

Sex is inevitably moist, smelly, and sweaty, and often involves bodies that aren't perfectly clean. It uses various openings in each body, including the mouth. And it involves, or is near, the excretory organs that process our daily waste products. Every ten-year-old knows how extremely gross the whole idea seems. To enjoy sex, you have to look at it entirely differently.

While most people don't go out of their way to make sex messier than necessary, a couple can choose to agree that sex is a place where the normal rules of decorum don't apply. You and your partner can decide that wetting the bed, drooling, grunting, and crying are acceptable, needing neither apology nor explanation. Making sex a "no-vigilance zone" can make it a lot easier to relax and let your body do what it wants, which is a pretty dependable way to increase pleasure, maintain self-esteem, and facilitate intimacy. Now *that's* Sexual Intelligence.

People who can't stand a mess find sex challenging, something to protect themselves from. Few people who need their partner to be squeaky clean (and to be clean themselves, of course) before consenting to sex can relax and enjoy it fully. And people who expect to remain clean and dry all the way through sex find it very difficult to enjoy. That's because they see bodies as a source of contamination, messiness, dirt, and unruliness, rather than a source of pleasure. They see the body as a problem rather than as a toy.

So when patients who complain about sex use words like *messy, sloppy, gushing, drooling, unclean, dirty,* or *disorganized,* I assess their tolerance for messes and bodies in general. I tell too-neat people that I'm sympathetic about how they're probably making sex more difficult than necessary. If their partner is in therapy with them, I remind them both not to take the other's preferences and needs as personal criticism or selfishness. And I encourage them to take a minute before they start sex to relax together and focus on the parts of each other's body that they like. Visualizing pleasure, calmness, and connection during sex is often helpful for the person concerned with the messiness of sex. I suggest that people learn to interpret the moisture and mess of sex as an expression of intimacy and safety rather than chaos and danger.

Trusting Your Own Body

Your body feels how it feels. Sometimes it gets excited. Sometimes it doesn't. Do you trust its judgment?

Our bodies have no morality other than immediate sensation. Your finger doesn't know if you're putting it in a socially "clean" part of your partner's body or a "dirty" part; your tongue doesn't know if you're licking a "normal" part of someone's body or a "kinky" part.

If we judge our physical experiences through a cultural filter—this is sex, this isn't, this is clean, this is dirty, this is normal, this is sick, this is gay—we deny the body its unmediated, uncivilized, raw intelligence and perception. We also keep sex a controlled, left-brain activity, whereas Sexual Intelligence suggests we can more easily enjoy it via the right brain. Unfortunately, some people have to think, during sex, about each caress, each kiss, each moment, before "deciding" whether to enjoy it and allow it to continue, or to reject it—as too kinky, too ambiguous, too dirty or nasty.

Note that this decision is different from "Yes, I want to have sex, and I don't like how that particular activity feels." Instead, this is "I can't allow myself to like this because of what I've decided it *means*." Over the years I've seen men who wouldn't let their wives kiss their nipples because "that's what gay guys are into"; I've seen women refuse to give their boyfriend a hand job because "I should use my vagina for that"; I've seen both men and women reject a friendly, moist finger near their anal opening because "that's way too kinky." Not "it hurts," or even "it will hurt," but "it's too kinky."

It's a little like facing a new food while traveling. Some people try the new food and judge it based on how it tastes. Others ask what it is and decide whether or not to try it based on how it sounds. "Dandelion buds? Flowers are made to look at, not eat." "Alligator? That can't be good." "A squash six feet tall? That's just too creepy." You miss a lot of life's richness that way.

If you're trying to keep everything in life from flying out of control, it's very hard to enjoy your body's anarchy (unless you've decided that sex is the one place where it's safe to let things go). Of course, the fear of losing control isn't always about sex—for many people it's part of a bigger unconscious neurotic project. Sex therapists see a lot of, um, control freaks. These patients often tell us how to do the therapy, how to rearrange the furniture, and why we should change the music in the waiting room. They often want to argue about the answer—and then complain that we're wasting their time.

Boundaries

Enjoyable sex requires that we invite the violation of our personal boundaries and accept that we're going to breach someone else's boundaries. Of course, that's part of what demands and facilitates intimacy in sex.

Much of sex involves putting a part of your body inside of someone else's body—a tongue, a finger, a penis; a mouth, a vagina, an anus. For some people, this voluntary, temporary violation of personal space is what sex is all about. But if you're not comfortable with this, the firmest erection or most luxuriant lubrication won't be worth much.

Are you emotionally present enough and comfortable enough to provide useful feedback to your partner while this is happening? If not, how can he or she possibly know what your experience is like? Some people like words, while others like gestures. Still others imagine that the psycho-erotic fusion is so complete that each partner just intuits the other's experience. (Sounds like being stoned back in the sixties.) For a grown-up in the twenty-first century, actual communication is your best bet.

But some people are extremely inhibited about expressing themselves. They imagine that their experience should not be acknowledged, or that the very expression of it is unattractive or inappropriate (which is like saying, "I want to make complete sentences, but I try to do so without 'k' and 'g' because they're so un-lady-like").

Some people hesitate to communicate during sex because genuine expression renders them vulnerable, which is scary. They're right—someone's more likely to know how you feel when you express yourself. As a therapist, I investigate what exactly makes this troublesome: Does experiencing pleasure contradict someone's self-image of being demure or wholesome? Does feeling *anything* sexual conflict with someone's self-image? There's something missing from sex without actual communication. What could explain such inhibition?

One thing that makes the boundary violation in (consensual) sex more comfortable is being confident that it will end when sex ends—the way serious competition in weekend tennis is okay if we're certain that it will end after the match. We lob the ball up high if our opponent is facing into the sun, but after the match we don't toss their car keys into the bushes, out of reach.

If personal boundaries are not respected *outside* sex, however, it's hard to choose to lower boundaries *within* sex. In fact, if there isn't a healthy division of power in a relationship, sex might be the one place where someone gives him- or herself permission to say no. Of course, sometimes people do this indirectly, via having a headache, picking a fight, being too tired, or taking on extra projects.

Salvadore's trauma had very little to do with sex. In order to divorce him and marry someone else decades ago, his ex-wife falsely accused him of assault, got a court order banishing him from their kids' lives, and then took all their money. He was so grief-stricken by this, and exhausted from endless rounds of lawyers, social workers, and psychiatrists, that he eventually lost his job, too. He withdrew from people in general, and from women in particular.

Three years ago he got involved with Elizabeth, an obese, lonely woman tired of living alone. One thing she wanted was sex. Another was touching. Salvadore, sixty-two years old at the time, couldn't deliver much of either. So Elizabeth brought them in for "sex therapy," essentially to fix him. In our initial sessions, Salvadore could barely look at me. Elizabeth complained about a lot of things: his clothes were old and didn't fit, he needed a haircut, he mumbled, he was sloppy around the house, and so on.

These observations were all true, but Elizabeth's continual criticism reminded Salvadore of his ex-wife, who had complained for years about how inept he was. On top of that, just being in a relationship reminded Salvadore of being married, which itself made him terribly anxious.

Never a person overly interested in touching or sexuality, Salvadore was just too traumatized to trust and relate to a partner, and his physical expressions of affection and even his physical presence simply collapsed under the emotional stress. As we soon uncovered, he had eventually coped with his ex-wife's threats and the endless aggressive interviews by police and social workers back then by dissociating. His mind just shut down his conscious psychological function, disrupting the normal processing of outside stimuli, distancing his mind from experiences that were too much for his psyche to handle.

Indeed, one of the reasons he did so poorly with judges and social workers was his inability to advocate on his own behalf, and his defeated, depressive body language and poor personal grooming supported his ex-wife's claim that he was unsuited for parenting.

Salvadore was literally traumatized. In fact, I diagnosed with him PTSD—post-traumatic stress disorder. Even though sex wasn't involved in the origin of his PTSD, his condition was creating sexual problems.

Because of his past marital nightmare, he frequently dissociated with Elizabeth, often without warning. When he did feel anything, it was typically rage. That would trigger her rage—she had her own problems with anger, and working on a high-pressure assembly line in a dysfunctional factory didn't help things. They'd fight a lot. Passive Salvadore would become Mean Salvadore. Neither Salvadore could function in a relationship or enjoy sex.

When dissociated, of course, Salvadore could barely touch Elizabeth and couldn't possibly make love—which drove her crazy. Sometimes he'd respond to her begging or bullying and caress her in a perfunctory way, or even acquiesce to passive sex. But of course she wanted much, much more.

his PTSD + her desire = relationship trouble

Before Salvadore could feel more desire for sex or even touch, therapy was going to be about welcoming Salvadore's body back into his life and into their relationship. So there were a few things we would need to do first. Our work had to include:

- Identifying Salvadore as struggling with PTSD

- Understanding the meaning of "dissociation" and its impact

- Elizabeth's recognition that Salvadore wasn't rejecting her personally

- Salvadore's recognition of what it was like for Elizabeth to be with someone whose body was missing from the relationship

- Helping them both see that neither of them was to "blame"

- Getting him to accept physical pleasure from *non*-physical activities

- Understanding that no matter how Elizabeth seemed at a given moment, she was *not* Salvadore's ex-wife

- Elizabeth's need to back way off—and not because her appetite for him was bad

- Structured touching exercises

- Both Salvadore and Elizabeth learning to recognize the symptoms of him disappearing emotionally—and learning how to stop sex if that happened, and to talk about it

After about a dozen very painful sessions, Salvadore sort of woke up from his trance. "Elizabeth's not perfect, but she's not my ex-wife, is she?" We all agreed that she wasn't. "So I don't have to protect myself from her?" he speculated cautiously.

For the first time in their entire relationship, he talked about experiences of "just turning off, shutting down, and going into suspended animation inside." He said the pain—the betrayal by his wife, the loss of his children, the humiliating and frightening interrogations by "cops and shrinks"—was so intense that it was just easier to "feel nothing, want nothing, be nothing."

This was the man whom Elizabeth wished would feel desire, feel pleasure, feel intimacy, and feel connected with his body. This was, sadly, completely unrealistic for Salvadore as he was. But he was motivated to change. So we started small. We're still working on it.

Experience and Comfort with Masturbation

A century ago, Oscar Wilde famously said, "To love oneself is the beginning of a life-long romance."

Masturbation is the ultimate example of this. In Western countries, over 90 percent of men and two-thirds of women masturbate at some point. In 2009, various European countries even started encouraging it as a healthy habit.

Of course not everyone feels the same about it. When my patients discuss it with me, I ask if they enjoy it. Many look at me like I'm crazy—"Of course I enjoy it, Doc, why else do it? Sheesh." But a sizable minority don't—they masturbate, but they feel guilty, selfish, or unfaithful (to spouse or even God), they rush so they won't get caught, they lie to their mates about it, or they feel frustrated when they don't climax.

The experience of masturbation is a vital part of Sexual Intelligence. While it isn't necessary for people to masturbate in the present in order to enjoy partner sex, it does help if they've done it at some point. Or if they never have, it's important that guilt, fear, or shame isn't the reason why.

Years (or decades) before partner sex, masturbation provides familiarity with your own body and with the feelings of desire, arousal, excitement, and satisfaction. Perhaps most importantly, it develops your *sexual agency,* the knowledge that:

- Your sexuality belongs to you.

- You can experiment with it without knowing exactly what will happen.

- You can create experiences that please you.

- Focusing on yourself sexually doesn't make you selfish or greedy, lewd or oversexed, or less than or different than you "really" are.

Contrast sexual agency with the idea that many children learn and often carry forward into adulthood: that the desire to masturbate is shameful or pathological, a sick impulse that must be resisted—one that will hurt them if they give in to it.

There's one more thing about sexual agency to remember—you can masturbate even when you're in a sexual relationship with someone. In fact, you can even masturbate if your partner complains about not getting enough sex with you. Of course, such a complaint should not be ignored, but in my clinical experience, masturbating less doesn't usually increase desire for one's partner. That's like saying, "Eat less ice cream, so you'll eat more broccoli." It rarely works; depriving your partner of a favorite sexual outlet typically doesn't increase her or his hunger for you.*

The next logical step of sexual agency is openly touching yourself *during* sex with a partner. How's that for challenging a taboo?

I'm not aware of any statistics about how many men and women do this, but I know it's not common. That's too bad, because there are so many good reasons to do it. Of course, pleasure is the first one. There's nothing like getting touched perfectly—the right speed, pressure, angle, location. And if you're really excited—say, from sexual activity with your partner—that might be just the time to take over and give yourself what you want. I don't call this masturbation, because masturbation is what you do when you're alone. I call this touching-yourself-during-partner-sex. That's more accurate, it sounds sexier, and it helps people overcome their inhibitions about it.

Of course, there are other reasons to touch yourself during partner sex. For example, it's the best way to show your partner what you like. If you're a woman, your male partner can't know just how

---

*When dealing with desire discrepancies or complaints about pornography use, many therapists make this same mistake—insisting that the low-desire partner stop masturbating in order to increase his or her desire for partner sex. If you can actually get someone to masturbate less (uncommon in my clinical experience), it rarely accomplishes anything. See Appendix 1 (written for and about professionals) for details.

sensitive your clitoris gets when you're really excited, or just what angle you want a finger to enter your vagina. If you're a man, you've known for years that women need instruction in how tightly (and when and where) to squeeze your balls.

The option of touching yourself during partner sex multiplies your possibilities. Four hands, not two. Angles and pressure not otherwise available. And it means you're not dependent on your partner's stamina—or interest. Your partner may swear that he or she will stay engaged after climaxing, but, well, sometimes that old post-orgasm-disengagement hormone kicks in, and then it's really good to lend yourself a hand. And if you're someone who enjoys (or needs) steady stimulation for a long time in order to climax, it's great to give your partner a break now and then (or, to think about it differently, for him or her to give you a break).

Finally, touching yourself during partner sex encourages your partner to do the same. If your partner has never done it, or feels too shy to even think about it, this will change his or her life. If you're already doing it, I'm guessing it changed yours, right?

The Gift of Staying Present

Some people don't realize that to enjoy sex, you have to pay attention. It isn't like TV, where you can just go on automatic pilot and let it happen. Well, I suppose you can just go on automatic during sex if you don't mind having sex that's like watching TV.

Many people don't actually know how to pay attention during sex.

It's a skill, like focusing on how something tastes (instead of reading or talking on the phone while you eat and missing the actual experience of the food), or on how enjoyable a movie is (instead of focusing on your uncomfortable seat), or on how beautiful the Golden Gate Bridge is (instead of getting irate about the miserable traffic).

There are many choices of what to attend to during sex. Listening for the people next door? Wondering if your stomach is getting bigger? Thinking maybe you should have showered first? Noticing that the drapes need dusting? Noticing that your husband needs dusting?

Of course, there's always the past to attend to: what it was like last time, what it was like the first time, what it was like two years ago, what about that time you farted during sex and your boyfriend teased you so much you thought you'd never get over it, what about that time you thought he was cheating on you and you had sex with him anyway for weeks afterwards even though you hated it. . . .

As William Faulkner once wrote, "The past is never dead. It's not even past."

And as we've seen elsewhere, their own sexual response is something that too many people attend to during sex: Am I getting excited enough? Excited enough fast enough? Erection okay? Lubrication okay? Have an orgasm? Time it takes to orgasm okay? That's a lot to think about. And it makes it harder to pay attention to how things look, taste, smell, sound, and feel. Which is where sex actually is experienced.

For some people, consciously inhabiting their body is scary. Having a quiet mind is scary. Paying attention to the input from fingertips, nose, and eyes feels too . . . too . . . *personal*. Too private. Sex with the body, sex with the quiet mind, paying attention during sex, for some people it just feels too intimate. All you have is you and the other person, with nothing to mediate or dilute the experience. And then worries about "maybe my balls are too hairy" or "I hope the shoe repair place is open on Sunday" are a welcome distraction.

If that sounds like you, I encourage you to stop the sex when you realize you're having trouble being present—yes, right in the middle—look at your partner, and gently say either:

- "Honey, can we slow down and start again?" or

- "Um, I'm not really in the mood like I thought I was. Maybe let's try again another time."

Add these phrases to your sexual vocabulary, and use when appropriate.

Focus your attention on how your body feels during sex. In fact, you could paint that on your bedroom ceiling.

The question is, when it comes to sex, is the body a problem to be tolerated, outwitted, and thwarted, or is it a resource, a toy, a locus of pleasure, a place of integrity? If it's the former, it will be hard to stay present, hard to connect with your partner (and his or her body), and hard to use your body to express positive sentiments or explore the self.

If it's the latter, all things are possible. Part of the job of therapy is helping people discover which experience of the body they're closer to, decide where they want to be, and figure out how to get there.

Part Three

Implications
and
Applications

Chapter Seven

Letting Go

Obstacles to Developing Sexual Intelligence

Winchester was a pretty nice guy—friendly bowler, cooperative husband, dependable dentist. No one in his life would describe him as stubborn—except me.

He originally came to me because he had lost much of his sexual desire and his erections were becoming less and less reliable. He loved his wife and really wanted their relationship, and sex life, to work. He described her as pretty, easygoing, and interested in sex.

"I just want sex to be the way it was," he said plainly. "I love Janie, and I want us to have a normal sex life again." Not unreasonable, I thought.

Winchester had been bowling almost every Monday for twenty years, with an impressive 220 average. But as with all sports, long-term, high-performance bowling had taken its toll on his body. He developed back pain in his late thirties, and it never went away. Year by year, it just got worse—a dull throb that became a sharp stab when he turned or bent the wrong way. As it happened, "the wrong way" included missionary position intercourse and getting on his knees to pleasure his wife orally.

That's right: sex hurt. Almost every time—sometimes a little, sometimes a lot. The pain demanded that he limit the positions in which he had intercourse or oral sex. But remember, Winchester was stubborn; so he kept making love in his favorite positions, withstanding increasingly frequent stabs of pain. Eventually, he would lose his erection at those times. And eventually he began to avoid sex.

He didn't want to admit this to Janie. We discussed his refusal to discuss this with her for many sessions, during which he acknowledged that she'd probably be sympathetic. "But I don't want sympathy," he complained. "I want to get on top of her and do her. Like a man."

"Apparently," I said quietly, "you can't have that. You can have a lot of sexual treasures in your life, but apparently not that one."

He was devastated. "I can never have good sex again?" "Yes, you can," I replied. "But not the way you think it's supposed to be." Most people think it's only women who sometimes experience painful sex. That's not accurate.

"Winchester," I said, "this isn't a sex problem so much as a spiritual or existential one. Only forty-four years old, you're being confronted by your own mortality. You're being forced to reinvent what it means to be a man."

Winchester would be forced to "settle"—unless he could be creative and reinvent sex and himself. It's something we're all challenged to do sooner or later. Some people succeed, others fail; many refuse to try, withdrawing into bitterness, depression, or solipsism. I told Winchester I was certain he could do the work of reinventing sex and masculinity for himself. He was, he finally confessed, frightened. "Of succeeding or failing?" He wasn't sure.

It took months. He worked through a bunch of stuff.

Toward the end of our work, he asked if he could bring in his wife. I was curious about her, of course. I'm always curious about the person who lives offstage in the drama of psychotherapy with a married person. But this was no time for indulging my curiosity—alas, there never is.

"Why do you want to bring her in?"

"So you can explain what we've discussed, and she can understand that I'm not just being a pussy."

"You have to do that," I said. "You don't need me, and you shouldn't have me do it."

"Why?"

"Because part of growing up is sitting her down and telling her exactly who you are right now. It's time to reach out to her and for you to lead the two of you through things collaboratively. You can do it."

"It's easier if you do it."

"Yes, you're right. But this isn't about doing what's easier. Sometimes sex is a vehicle for growing up, which is never the easiest option. It's often the best, although not necessarily the easiest."

So he told her. They made a decision—no more missionary position sex. They both cried—she was losing something too. "But I don't want sex that hurts you," she said. "And any sexual connection with you is way better than nothing. Way, way better."

* * *

Sexual Intelligence is about focusing on the right things before, during, and after sex. But part of Sexual Intelligence is also about knowing what to let go of. Obviously, focusing on the wrong things makes it harder to focus on the right things.

So let's actually name some common things on which people focus, and explain the importance of letting these things go. Then in the next chapters we can talk explicitly about what to focus on instead, and how.

Being "Normal"

This is an easy place to start, because we already took a long look at this issue all the way back in Chapter 2.

So this is just a reminder: my goal is *not* to reassure you that "even if you're different, you're normal." No, my agenda is more ambitious: I want you to forget about the question of normality altogether.

I know that's challenging, because it means claiming your own power to evaluate your sexuality, rather than getting the reassurance of comparing yourself to others. So how would letting go of this idea of sexual normality change things? Here's one way: If you completely let go of it, wouldn't you feel closer to your partner? Might there be something you'd be willing to ask or discuss with him or her about sex?

I'm betting there is. And that has to be good for your sex life.

So I propose that you Let It Go.

Intercourse

Penis-vagina intercourse is what most people call "real sex."

If you're old enough to remember life before the Internet, you'll recall the bizarre Monica Lewinsky scandal, which seemed to last a lifetime. It climaxed with President Bill Clinton swearing, before TV camera, wife, and God, that "I did not have sexual relations with that woman."

It turned out he was being literal—"sexual relations" has long been a euphemism for penis-vagina intercourse, which he apparently did *not* have with "that woman."

But of course he did other things that most people think of as sex. And so people accused Clinton of lying. He later apologized on national television for deliberately misleading people—underlining, however, that he had been legally accurate.

So whassup with intercourse? Why do I diss going all the way, hiding the salami, jumping someone's bones, getting laid, fornicating, boinking, laying pipe, riding the love machine, shtupping, knocking boots, burying the bone, going to the drive-in, doing the horizontal mambo, effing, humping, nailing, hammering, pounding, drilling, porking, plowing, shagging, or screwing?

Okay, let us count the ways. The disadvantages of intercourse include:

- It's the only kind of sex that requires an erection.

- It's the only kind of sex that requires birth control.

- It's not an especially effective way for most women to orgasm.

- It can be painful for women in middle age and beyond, and therefore painful for their partners, too.

- It's an especially easy way to transmit diseases.

- It can be hard to fit the body parts together without looking at them (especially if you don't talk much about doing so, either before or while you're trying).

- It isn't necessarily intimate (so quit using the word *intimacy* to mean *sex* or *intercourse*).

- It generally doesn't get you excited if you aren't already excited.

But the big problem isn't actually with intercourse itself. It's with our *relationship* to intercourse—the belief that it's the only "real sex," the feeling that everything else is "foreplay" (the second-rate stuff before intercourse), and the belief that once we get excited we need to "go all the way" in order to be successful and satisfied. This constricted view limits our flexibility, and is the exact opposite of what most people say they want from sex—playfulness, spontaneity, ease.

While much of this would be true no matter what else we might decide is "real sex," making intercourse the Number One Special Sexual Activity creates the extra problem that "real sex" always carries the risk of unwanted conception.

If you don't assume that all sex will end with intercourse, you can:

- Begin sexual activity without having to worry about your "function"

- Enjoy erotic activity without the distraction of monitoring "where it's going"

- Focus on the activities you like rather than focusing on getting increasingly excited

So I propose that you Let It Go.

A Hierarchy of Sexual Activities

For most adults, cultural competency around sex includes a hierarchy: everyone knows that some sexual activities are somehow superior or more like "real sex" than others. Note that being "more like real sex" is *not* the same thing as being "more enjoyable." People may disagree about which things are better than which, but most adults do believe in some sort of sexual hierarchy.

Different American cultures and ethnic groups value different aspects of sexuality, including, for example, modesty, experimentation, self-control, refusing contraception, multiple partners, being pain-free, female submission, the act of seduction, and orgasm itself. Nevertheless, the consensus in Western culture is that the pinnacle of the heterosexual hierarchy is intercourse. This means, depending on who you ask, that intercourse is the sexual activity that is the most "serious," the most dangerous, the most enjoyable, the most intimate, the most godly, the most "natural," or the most "normal."

Most Americans would agree that right below intercourse is other genital sex with a partner (such as oral sex, anal sex, and hand jobs), followed by masturbation and non-genital sex. Kissing is a wild card, because for some people it's boring, intrusive, or a turnoff; for others, kissing is the height of intimacy. (You can have intercourse when you're angry, but kiss? Eeyew, gross!)

Commercial sex, Internet sex, phone sex, "alternative" or "kinky" sex (S/M, for example), fetishes (feet, urination, gloves, and so on)—each occupies a space of its own. For practitioners, these activities are very hot, while nonpractitioners usually just scratch their heads and say, "But where's the *sex* in it?"

So how does attention to this imagined hierarchy undermine our satisfaction?

Believing in a sexual hierarchy devalues our experience—people dismiss what they've done (or been offered) as "only foreplay" or "not real sex." The hierarchy can also make sex more complicated if partners disagree on the meaning of a certain activity. (For example, foot massage: sexy and intimate, or a not-sexy waste of time?)

A hierarchy introduces success and failure into sexual decision-making and experience; if you judge your sexual adventure as insufficiently high up on the ladder, you may feel cheated or self-critical. Similarly, a hierarchy introduces the idea of "dysfunction": if there's something you need to do to be sexually "successful," that creates the category of "unable to do the thing to be successful"—i.e., dysfunction.

Deciding that it's intercourse at the peak of the hierarchy, of course, brings its own special problems: the possibility of pregnancy, along with the requirement of an erect penis and a lubricated vagina. Overvaluing intercourse also encourages us to overfocus on orgasm, and it demeans self-touch with a partner instead of allowing us to see it as one of many equal erotic choices.

Sexual Intelligence involves knowing that our familiar sexual hierarchy is just a cultural artifact, and that we aren't required to be loyal to it. For example, as Shere Hite documented forty years ago, men's and women's strongest orgasms are typically from masturbation, not partner sex; and for women, most orgasms occur from clitoral stimulation, not intercourse. Even though their own experience attests to this truth, many people ignore this and attempt to do sex the mythical "right way"—and get frustrated with the results.

Since the whole hierarchy is arbitrary, we shouldn't be surprised when it changes over time. The cultural meaning of, say, cunnilingus has changed dramatically over the last one hundred years. The experience of losing one's virginity is often quite different now than it was fifty years ago. And the meaning, incidence, and place in the hierarchy of anal sex have changed dramatically in just twenty-five years.

Of course, since the hierarchy is built on arbitrary social norms, any given activity may have more symbolic value than practical value for someone. That is, you may feel you should enjoy something more than you do, or you may choose to do something when you don't especially enjoy it. (This may be especially true if, like many people today, you're watching more porn.) Examples might include anal play, "tit fucking," and intercourse itself—activities valued by some people more for what they represent than for the amount of pleasure they actually offer.

When two people have sex, it's hard enough for them to find common interests, get their bodies to do what they want them to do, and find the time, energy, and privacy to do it. Caring too much about which activities are "right" or somehow acceptable makes sex—and life—way too complicated. We're much better off discovering what we like, learning how to create it, and getting comfortable with instructing others on our preferences. Which kind of sex is better than which other kind of sex? Those old hierarchies are for accountants, not lovers.

So what about oral sex? A hand job? Phone sex? Masturbating during an Internet chat session? Going to a strip club? Reading a romance novel and getting excited? Over the years I've had many patients argue over whether they'd just been caught having "an affair," or doing something they claimed was far less important. "That's not sex, that's typing," said one woman defending her chat-room escapades. It reminded me of what Truman Capote said decades ago about Jack Kerouac's book *On the Road*: "That's not writing, that's typing."

So I propose that you Let It Go.

Performance Obsession—The Agony of Failure, the Anxiety of Success

For some people, not failing is the best that sex ever gets. This is especially true of many young people, before they've established their internal sense of sexual identity and adequacy.

We can all do better than that.

Many men and women come into my office wanting help with this, saying things like: "My performance isn't so good," or, "I'm about to start sleeping with this new guy, and given my ugly last relationship, I want to make sure my performance doesn't disappoint him."

Why turn sex into a performance? It doesn't start out that way—we *make* it that way through our vision. It's similar to the way some people turn drinking into a performance—they brag about drinking more than everyone else, or tease others about not being able to hold their liquor. I recall a patient who bragged, "I could drink a table under the table," which I guess is a lot. Meanwhile, other people think drinking is just drinking.

Imagine if we did this with, say, eating broccoli: "Wow, that guy can put away more broccoli than anyone. And not even fart afterwards. What a man!" Or: "Hey, Mary could hardly down a single stalk of broccoli last week. I bet she won't be showing her face around here for a while!"

Constantly monitoring your performance not only erodes your enjoyment of sex, it also makes it harder to "perform" the way you want to. That's because, in real life, "performance" isn't voluntary; it's part of the autonomic nervous system, the body's uncontrollable response to stimuli, both internal and external. If you're paying attention to your desire to perform (or your terror about failing to do so), it's that much harder to feel, smell, touch, and taste the body you're with, or to see that person smile.

Not surprisingly, our culture's emphasis on performance has made erection drugs enormously successful. Also not surprisingly, more and more young men *without* erection problems are using these drugs. Over the years, I've had a few dozen patients under twenty-five tell me, "It's just for insurance. If there's a good chance I'll be hooking up, I take it. Nobody has to know, and there's no harm done."

Well, it's not as bad for you as shooting heroin, but I actually do think there's harm done. Specifically, young guys who take Viagra-type drugs when they don't need them never get to find out they don't need them. They don't get to build their confidence, because when they get the adequate erections they desire, they credit the drug. Some guys say that this effect is in fact what's building their confidence and that eventually they'll stop taking the drug, but I haven't seen that a whole lot since the drug became popular over a decade ago.

There's also the secrecy that develops—these guys rarely tell their partners they're using an erection drug, and the more they use it the bigger the secret becomes. And while that isn't as bad as shooting heroin either, I've never seen a relationship that needed more secrets.

Some psychologists say that people attend to their performance as a way of maintaining psychological distance with a partner. Or that they're so narcissistic that their real erotic object is their own body and its performance, rather than their partner. Perhaps that's true. Whether people do this to create the distance or simply accept the distance that results (or don't even notice it) is an open question—but emotional distance is rarely a good thing.

It's ironic: people focused on performance typically say, "I want to give my partner a good time," or, "I don't want to disappoint my partner." Then they emotionally withdraw from their partner to pursue their own agenda of creating a sexual performance they feel proud of, rather than being emotionally present, which most people prefer in a partner.

So I propose that you Let It Go.

"Function" and "Dysfunction"

Too many people think that if your penis or vulva does tricks when and how you want, you "function" right, and that if not, you have a "dysfunction."

Most people stuck on this model don't seem to appreciate the role of emotion in facilitating or blocking sexual "function." We get erect or wet (genitally, I mean) as the result of an impressive chain of events:

- Our brain perceives a sexual message (for some, a photo of Bristol Palin; for others, that's the end of erections for a month).

- Our brain sends a message down the spinal column toward the pelvic nerves.

- The pelvic nerves send a message to the small blood vessels radiating out from the pelvis.

- The blood vessels receive the message and get to work: they dilate, allowing more blood to flow in.

- The increased blood flow fills the penis or clitoris, making it hard, and triggers the wetness that eventually sweats through the vaginal wall into the vagina.

How the Mind/Body Creates Sexual Arousal

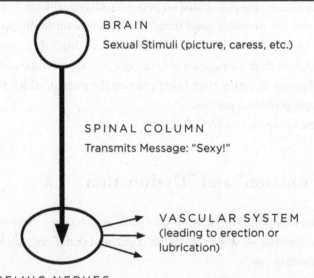

BRAIN
Sexual Stimuli (picture, caress, etc.)

SPINAL COLUMN
Transmits Message: "Sexy!"

VASCULAR SYSTEM
(leading to erection or lubrication)

PELVIC NERVES
Instructs Blood Vessels

It's a very cool process when it works. But obviously, a lot can go wrong: a problem with the information transfer between brain and spinal column, between spinal column and pelvic nerves, or between pelvic nerves and blood vessels; the nonresponsiveness of the blood vessels once they do get the message; or the disruptions created by diseases like diabetes, high blood pressure, arteriosclerosis, and Alzheimer's, as well as by spinal cord injuries (from sports, car accidents, military injuries, and so on).

There's another possible problem: the spinal column also carries our emotions, which are basically simple electrical impulses (I know, a hopelessly romantic point of view). Note that the message "Alert—sexual excitement, prepare for pelvic hydraulics!" is carried down the same pipe as the message "I don't trust you, mister," or, "You still haven't apologized to my mother," or, "What the hell am I doing here?" These emotions serve as noise, which can prevent a clean sexual signal from getting all the way to the pelvis from the brain. The result? Not enough signal to create vasocongestion down there, or to keep it flowing after it starts. You know that old Bulgarian saying: inadequate vasocongestion, inadequate "function."

"Sexual dysfunction" is when the brain–spinal column–pelvic nerves–vascular system information transfer doesn't work smoothly.

A high percentage of people who come to see me with "sexual dysfunction" are experiencing emotional noise while they're expecting a sexual message to get them or keep them aroused. That's not sexual dysfunction; that's the body working fine, just contrary to its owner's wishes.

Think of it this way: if you eat at McDonald's three times a day for a month, sooner or later you're going to get a serious stomachache. When you go to the doctor with awful cramps, the first question will be: "What have you been eating?" When you tell the truth (proudly or shamefaced), the doctor will say, "Oh, good news— your stomach works fine. Your stomach isn't *designed* to digest

McDonald's food smoothly three times a day for a month. So your pain is a sign that your stomach is working perfectly. Now go away and start eating broccoli."

It's the same thing with your penis or vulva. When you're metaphorically eating at McDonald's three times a day—when you're filled with a lot of anger, sadness, loneliness, confusion, or shame—your body isn't supposed to be able to get and stay hot. This is true whether you're aware of those feelings or not, or whether you admit them to yourself or not. If you're making love with a new friend and she suddenly says, "Omigod, I think I hear my husband coming up the stairs," you're definitely going to lose your erection. That isn't erectile dysfunction—you're not *supposed* to be able to keep an erection in such a situation. At that point, your body needs the blood for more important things—like propelling itself out the window.

So I propose that you Let It Go.

The Need for a Perfect Environment for Sex

Consider Paris, a very special place. Anyone can enjoy it if they have plenty of money, the weather is great, and they speak French. Since any given trip to Paris may lack one, two, or all three of these, however, the trick is to be able to enjoy Paris without them.

Many people are capable of wanting and enjoying sex under the perfect conditions: the right partner; two perfectly clean bodies; complete privacy (I knew a patient so shy, she would only make love during a total eclipse of the sun, when there wouldn't be light anywhere within a thousand miles); not a single chore to do (I had a patient once who made her kids promise to wash the dishes and do the laundry immediately if they ever found her dead); no quarrels with their mate in at least six years; and both partners having gone to the gym *and* flossed that very day.

In other words, practically never. Maybe even never again.

Adults live complicated lives, and there are no time-outs. Therefore, if we want to enjoy sex, we will almost always do so under less-than-ideal conditions. That doesn't mean we don't have preferences and even have-tos; of course we do.

For some people, their have-to is brushing teeth; for others it's not having sex during their period, and for still others sex can't happen when they have a sinus headache or their back is out. I've known patients who couldn't have sex on an empty stomach, or while country music was playing, or with a pet in the room. I've also had patients who insisted on having their pet in the room during sex. Even exhibitionists are a heterogeneous group.

But think of this as an opt-in versus opt-out situation. Assuming our basic conditions are met, we need to be leaning toward yes unless there's a problem—rather than leaning toward no unless a long list of conditions is filled and a long list of deal-breakers is absent. If you're oriented toward reasons that you can't have sex on a given occasion rather than reasons that you can, you will benefit from enhancing your Sexual Intelligence.

A special note for parents: if you can't learn how to enjoy sex with kids in the house (presumably asleep, although less so as they get older), you're doomed to eighteen or more years of no sex (unless, of course, you can afford boarding school for either them or you).

Some people are fine with this. But if you'll be continually grumbling to your mate or resentful of your kids, you should develop a repertoire of activities and vocal levels: sex-with-kids-in-house (sleeping), sex-with-kids-in-house (awake), and sex-with-kids-not-in-house. For some people, there's also sex-with-spouse-not-in-house, but that's a different story entirely.

So I propose that you Let It Go.

The Need for "Spontaneity"
and Noncommunication

What adult does *anything* spontaneously anymore?

Let me put that another way: most of the spontaneity in adult life comes from good planning, deliberate maintenance of inventory, and a dependable system for doing things. Here are a few examples:

- *Going bike-riding:* Whether you plan ahead or do it spur-of-the-moment, you have to own a bike; know how to ride; have the right clothes for the weather (maybe you even check weather.com before you dress); put air in the tires; fill your water bottle (you do have one, right?); and bring your chain and lock (and don't forget the key). Whew, I'm half-exhausted just thinking about it. Well, if you do all this, then you can bike anywhere you like, for as long as you like. If your clothes match the weather, that is.

- *Going on a picnic:* The week before, we divide up who's going to bring food, drinks, a blanket, a Frisbee, and music. Then we can pursue these things in any order we like or even skip a few. But we can't do much that requires equipment we didn't bring.

- *Making chili for four:* After your bike ride or picnic, you feel generous and decide to invite people over for dinner. C'mon over this second, you say. Fortunately, you have a few essential ingredients for this gathering: you've stored some meat in the freezer; you have a microwave oven to defrost things; you cleaned up the kitchen last night; and you know how to cook. After you've shared half a bottle of chardonnay, you can decide when you're going to eat and whether vegetables will just ruin the mood.

- *Finally, making love:* When you get into the bedroom—with a stop off at the bathroom first—you set up your temporary love-shack. You take out whatever supplies are appropriate: birth control, lubricant, disease protection, toys, leather and lace. Having talked about it, you know that showers won't be necessary. And you've discussed spanking (not for you), sharing fantasies about co-workers (not for your partner), and talking nasty (you both like it). Having done this planning (including that stop in the bathroom), having had a key conversation or two, now you can have "spontaneous" sex—you can do whatever activities you both desire, in any order you like. You can even skip "normal" sex if you want to.

You've heard that in some cases "less is more"? Well, when it comes to sex, "spontaneity" requires planning.

Whether you're thirty, fifty, or seventy, most people remember the "spontaneity" of sex in their early years. But let's take a closer look at these "memories."

First, it wasn't completely spontaneous—typically, one or both parties had been thinking about it night and day; one or both parties had been rehearsing how to make it happen, how to make it *seem* spontaneous, and how to dress just right for it (for example, looking available enough to keep a partner interested, but not so available as to be considered a slut). And in terms of repertoire, our first sex is rarely spontaneous, as many of us are trying to fit into preexisting categories: a real man, a woman in love, a tormented romantic soul, and so on.

That said, there often was a spontaneous side to our early sexual experiences: many of us were drunk or stoned, we often didn't think much about the implications (Do I call the next day? What does she think this means? Will we still be friends?), and perhaps we did very little about contraception or disease protection. In fact, if you could do it all over again, would you do your early sexual experiences exactly the same? Or would you prepare a bit more, communicate a bit better, give some more thought to birth control? How about a bit more light in the room? So much for the ideal of "spontaneity."

And of course, that early "spontaneous" sex often led to a certain amount of heartbreak. Heartbreak is an occupational hazard of new sexual experiences and relationships, of course, but some of them could have been avoided by a few honest, nonspontaneous words: "I've never done this before," "I haven't done this in a long time," "If we do this I want it to mean we're a couple," "I have herpes," "I usually don't orgasm with a new person, so don't take it personally," "I feel really self-conscious about my scar," "Let's agree that this is private and we won't tell anyone, okay?"

Some would argue that these mini-conversations (which rarely *feel* "mini," which is why we hesitate to have them) take the "romance" out of sex. I think that's just fine—who needs some spurious "romance" when you can have real sex in real life? There's so much mystery integral to our sexuality, so much romance in getting to know a new body and a new person (or enjoying familiar things we've learned to expect), that we really don't need to add more of either one by hesitating to communicate, plan, or acknowledge what we're doing.

I believe that when people say they want sex to be spontaneous, they're thinking one or more of the following:

- I don't want to think about what I'm doing.

- I don't want to think about the consequences of what I'm doing.

- I don't want to be that close to the person I'm doing this with.

- I'm concerned that if either of us thinks about this, we won't do it.

- I'm concerned that talking about what we're doing will make it less interesting.

- I'm concerned that if I think too much about it my body won't "function."

I'm sympathetic about concerns like these, although my response to all of them is the same: don't pursue a sexual situation that you're not comfortable with. Too many people, especially young people, treat sexual opportunity as if it were Halley's Comet—like it comes around so rarely that they should grab it when they can, even if that means doing it under less than ideal conditions—that is, "spontaneously."

No. Unless you're in the French Foreign Legion, sex comes around again.

The fact is, "spontaneous" (read: nonthinking, noncommunicative) sex has too many disadvantages:

- You may feel isolated or alone while it's happening.

- You may feel that your performance is the main thing you offer.

- Your partner may feel that their performance is the main thing they offer.

- It often means no lubricant, contraception, or disease consideration, and limited physical comfort.

- But most of all, you miss some of the best parts of sex: being present, having a partner who's present, directing what's happening, being conscious.

So I propose that you Let It Go.

The Idea That Sex Has
Inherent Meaning

Sex has no inherent meaning. We can make individual sexual experiences meaningful, and if we have enough of them, we can say that sex is meaningful to us. But sex is meaningless until and unless we give it meaning. This gives us a lot of responsibility and a lot of power.

That said, most people give sex too much meaning, and the wrong kind of meaning. Then they complain that sex is too complicated. And they're right—when we make sex complicated, it's, um, complicated. It makes each sexual encounter too, um, meaningful. There's too much riding on each occasion, which creates pressure and anxiety that undermine sex.

What are the typical meanings that various people and institutions claim sex has? I periodically hear people say that the meaning of, foundation of, or distinctive feature of human sexuality is:

- Intimacy

- A divine gift to humans, which should be expressed divinely

- A validation of our identities as men or women

- A way to strengthen the (holy, matrimonial) relationship

- The ultimate expression of love

- The ultimate gift to someone

- The source of life (via conception)

- What people do if they love each other

- The fulfillment of desire

To make things even more complicated, it's also common for people to believe that:

- Healthy sexual desire is driven primarily by love

- Healthy, mature people are driven to sexual exclusivity

It's bad enough that people give sex all these meanings—which are too complicated, and often contrary to experience. (Everyone's had sex that was not at all "intimate," and most couples have had sex that didn't nurture the relationship one bit.) Believing that these features are or should be inherent in sex just makes things worse—because when we experience sex that doesn't reflect these ideals, we assume there's something wrong with us or our partner.

So what's the difference between *believing* that sex has meaning and *giving* it meaning? Why does it matter?

If you believe that sex has inherent meaning, you inevitably want to have sex in ways that are likely to deliver that meaning. It's one more way of being loyal to sexual standards outside of yourself, and it's as far from "spontaneous" and "being yourself" as possible. Many people become concerned that they're not fulfilling some duty to "honor" sex (a common idea among those who believe that God has gifted us with our sexuality). It's part of America's obsession with not making love "like animals"—as if we do it in ways that are somehow superior to other creatures.

I don't think we should be serving sex; I think sex should serve each of us. Each sexual encounter is an opportunity for us to create sex anew for ourselves, to use it to refresh and explore ourselves in personally relevant ways. If we think that sex has inherent meaning, and that it's our job to both find and conform to that meaning, we won't be able to see sex freshly, we won't be motivated to perceive or act counterintuitively, and we'll accept arbitrary, outside limits on our erotic activities. If you tolerate sex becoming smaller, you will become smaller along with it.

If you want to give sex meaning, go ahead. At the same time, remember that you can enjoy the freedom of playful, amoral (not immoral, *amoral*) sex. As Woody Allen says, "Sex without love is meaningless, but as far as meaningless experiences go, it's pretty damn good."

Some social institutions purport to tell us what sex means or what it "should" embody. Most organized religion, for example, is highly involved in controlling and *limiting* people's sexual expression. In fact, American Christianity has institutionalized its sexual norms politically, in abstinence ("sex education") training, obscenity laws, and pharmacists' "conscience clauses." Be wary of those who claim to know what sex "means" or what its "purpose" is—they want to control you by explaining how you should adapt your sexual expression so it's right.

With the Sexual Intelligence perspective that sex has only *emergent* meaning, you can experience a huge range of sexual feelings and meanings. Without this perspective, however, much of this range is either invisible, or, worse, repugnant, and by definition excluded. It brings to mind Nietzsche's aphorism, "Those who danced were thought insane by those who couldn't hear the music." You and your partner have the human privilege of listening to your own sexual music and dancing to it in your own unique way.

Finally, some people are afraid that if sex has inherent meaning and they don't salute it, they won't behave ethically. This is a common idea of those involved with religion—that it's religion that makes people behave ethically, and that lack of religion would remove this ethical regulator. This is a terribly pessimistic view of people—that they behave well only because they've been promised a reward after they die, or they fear great punishment after they die.

That's how five-year-olds think—reward and punishment. As adults, we can do better than that.

So I propose that you Let It Go.

"I can't stop," he continued. "I keep doing it, I watch myself do it, I say, 'Dino, don't do it,' and I do it anyway. Maybe I'm a 'love addict.'"

There were several things keeping Dino stuck in this *Groundhog Day*–like recurring pattern. As we discussed over time, he had failed, as a child, to rescue his mother from his alcoholic father. Hmm, so rescuing women as an adult might be an unconscious attempt to rectify this childhood "failure." Another factor was his low self-esteem and the resulting low expectations; he would periodically joke about always ending up with women in trouble, because who else would be attracted to him?

The third factor that kept him trapped was his incredibly romantic vision of sexual relationships. He would throw around expressions like "soulmate," "the only one for me," "the chemistry uniting our spirits," and "our destiny to be together." Hanging on to concepts like these is asking for trouble. We get attached to the *idea* of the other person rather than seeing the *actual* person; we get attached to the *concept* of the relationship instead of noticing our actual relationship *experience*. It's one of the ways people end up staying in a relationship long after it's become destructive.

Finally, Dino needed every woman with whom he slept to judge him the best lover she'd ever had. This impossible goal was how he set himself up for failure, disappointment, humiliation, and self-loathing (in that predictable order). Sometimes he hadn't received this "certification" before realizing the relationship was doomed, pointless, or actually destructive; at that point he'd double his efforts to achieve sexual approval as soon as possible—thus keeping him in the relationship. As things deteriorated, with anger, mean words, or days of no contact, he'd become more desperate to get his acknowledgment. He just couldn't handle the possibility that a future ex-girlfriend might not say he had been the best.

While Dino admitted that he needed to change some of his ideas and hadn't been able to, he drew the line at his vision of sex and sexual relating. "Oh, no," he said. "I'm not giving up my romantic ideas about sex and love. And I can't accept not being the best. If I give those up, I have nothing. No, you can't persuade me on this."

So there we were: his ideas about sex were a key problem, and he didn't want to examine them, much less give them up. He instinctively feared that giving up his romantic, "best lover" ideas would change everything. I said I agreed—giving up these ideas might make him less eager to fall in love, less sure of himself, more introspective, even less relentlessly cheerful. And more adult.

Dino needed a major transfusion of self-discipline. Emotionally he was all over the place, cheerful about too many damn things (as if he weren't connected to the reality of any of them), and feeling powerless about practically everything.

I had a teacher who used to say that our patients behave as if they don't believe what they know. Dino *knew* that:

- He couldn't rescue his mother from his father back when he was growing up.

- This made him want to rescue every needy or stuck woman he met.

- Perceiving such relationships as deeply intimate, and investing energy, time, and money in them, would result in him feeling disappointed, frustrated, and self-critical.

So why did he abandon all discipline when faced with a pretty face? Because he was trying to address an emotional deficit that he preferred not to admit he had. He was using sex and romance to medicate something that had nothing to do with sex.

Over several months, we talked about what it would be like to give up his project of rescuing the women of the world. At first he didn't always take our work seriously, but when we kept coming back to his dark vision of worthlessness and shame, he began to see its importance. I was very sympathetic—what boy doesn't want to save his mother? What boy wouldn't feel bad about failing to do so? "And what boy," I said, looking at him very, very gently, "what boy could possibly succeed in that situation?"

"So I didn't fail?" he asked, tearfully. "You know, she really needed help."

"Yes," I said, "I understand she did. But no boy could have done it. You tried your hardest, I'm sure."

When his emotional wall finally cracked, the tears finally came. Decades of shame, self-hatred, and desperate loneliness flooded him. "I'm tired, so tired," he said. "Can I please rest? I don't want to help any more women for a while."

I wanted to give him permission so much. Instead, I said, "Dino, if you want to rest, you can decide to do that. You can even decide to end your rescue project altogether."

"It's okay?" he asked.

"Dino, you don't need to ask me. I'll support you no matter what you decide."

"I want to stop," he said. "I'm stopping. I'm done. I'm done!" he said almost defiantly.

It took several months for him to come to terms with the implications of his decision. He also had to wrap up a relationship in which he was *not* going to get the validation he wanted. "So I just go ahead and feel bad?" he asked.

"Yes," I smiled. "You just feel bad about the relationship not working out, about your affection not being returned, about your efforts not being appreciated. You don't have to do anything about it."

"This is both terrible and great," he said. And he was right.

* * *

Let's talk about some practical approaches to developing your Sexual Intelligence, such as communicating better, paying closer attention, and redefining "sexy."

Know Your Conditions

What are your conditions for good sex? Do you know how to create them? How often do you make love when you don't have the conditions you need?

In his classic 1978 book *Male Sexuality* (now available as *The New Male Sexuality*), Dr. Bernie Zilbergeld discussed the concept of conditions for good sex. He said that everyone has conditions, or requirements, for enjoying sex.

I believe that conditions can be divided into three categories: those about yourself, those about the environment, and those about your partner. Examples of conditions include:

- *About yourself:* You need to feel clean. You need to have no chores pending.

- *About the environment:* You need privacy. You need a softly lit, romantic room.

- *About your partner:* You need your partner to say, "I love you." You need your partner to be drop-dead gorgeous.

Many common conditions express cultural ideals. For example, some people can't enjoy sex if they believe that they can be heard. Thus, they can't make love at home unless their kids are gone; they also have trouble in hotels if they believe the walls are too thin. Other people can't enjoy sex unless the man initiates, or makes more money than the woman.

Some conditions are more unusual: Some people can only enjoy sex if the woman is wearing high heels or lingerie. Others require absolute silence or constant chatter, or the risk of being seen. Otherwise, sex is boring or scary.

We can all benefit from identifying and understanding what we need to enjoy sex. Then we can ask ourselves: Do our conditions fit our values? Do our conditions attract the kind of people and experiences we want? Or are our conditions so narrow that satisfaction is almost impossible? If you desire a sense of danger, for example, you'll be fine as long as you're with a partner who isn't hostile or self-destructive. Similarly, if you can't take pleasure in sex unless every single one of your chores is completed, you may never enjoy sex in this lifetime.

How do your conditions match with those of your partner? If you need a lot of time to feel connected and relaxed and your partner is impulsive or noncommunicative, it will be hard for you both to feel comfortable at the same time. Similarly, if you like nasty talk but your partner enjoys lots of soft words and gentle looks, it may be difficult to create an environment you both like.

Couples in such situations, unfortunately, often argue about who is right and who is "unreasonable," "uptight," or "kinky." This is not real communication.

Instead, people in such situations need to share their disappointment, anxiety, and self-criticism. If a couple can decide that neither partner's conditions are wrong, they can begin to strategize about how to make love in ways that satisfy them both: For instance, they can take turns getting their conditions met. Or they can interpret their conditions in new ways. For example, if privacy is an issue, playing music or wearing a blindfold during sex can provide a sense of sexy seclusion.

Similarly, instead of needing to be squeaky clean before making love, a talk with your partner about how he or she actually feels about your body smells may be helpful. And having your partner stroke your genitals with a damp towel may satisfy your need for cleanliness in a way that enhances the sexual mood rather than detracting from it.

Although Seamus had lived in the United States for over ten years, to me he sounded as if he'd walked in off the movie set of *Angela's Ashes* or *Michael Collins*. "Yes," he smiled, "I do have a bit of a brogue, don't I?"

Seamus's marriage, career, children, and house were here in California. His parents, sisters, friends, and favorite foods were in Dublin. He was torn in half, wanting to be loyal to both his lives. He was, as my Yiddish grandmother used to say, trying to dance at two weddings with one backside (it really sounds better if you say "tuchas" instead of "backside").

He wasn't handling the conflict too well.

Some years he visited Ireland three or four times, inevitably arguing with his wife Catherine about using their money to do so. On the other hand, whenever he spent one of the kids' school holidays in California, his mother would sigh, his father would frown, his sisters would complain, and he would feel awful.

So Seamus, with one eye on Ireland and one eye on his kids, became increasingly discontented. Catherine tried to help, to no avail. His kids wanted more of his attention. That didn't help. So did she. That really didn't help. In fact, over time he became less and less interested in sex, which was why she insisted he see me.

He told me about feeling split, ultimately resenting Catherine for "pressuring" him. I suggested it might be easier to resent someone five feet away than people five thousand miles away. "Maybe it's also easier to resent Catherine than to feel hopeless and guilty," I added gently.

"You don't understand," he said, shaking his head. "She's gained some weight since having the kids. The house is always a mess—she says she'd rather draw or sing with the kids than badger them to clean up their room. And she hates to cook. Half the time she asks me to pick up something on the way home, or we have some weird combination of stuff.

"These things add up," he said decisively. "Who can be in the mood for sex when everything's out of control?"

That must have been exactly how he felt—out of control.

And his house growing up in Ireland? "Ah, that was a home," he fairly glowed.

And that was his picture of how things ought to look now: "My father's house," he recalled with a lilt. "Everything's organized, everything revolves around him. Supper when he comes home. Quiet when he reads the paper. Kids answer when they're spoken to. Wife saying, 'Yes, dear,' when he's grumpy. No conflict, no wife saying, 'We don't communicate like we used to.'"

And, he added, "I certainly can't imagine my mum complaining about not having sex often enough!"

No, Catherine wasn't like his mum, and Seamus's California house wasn't like his dad's. It was messy, noisy, full of life. And it had a wife who rarely said, "Yes, dear," even when he was grumpy.

What about when they had courted? "She was the most colorful woman I'd ever met," he recalled. "I was fascinated."

Colorful she still was. But as she had grown, acquiring the responsibilities of a family and home, she had become more independent. Her "color" combined with her independence was difficult for Seamus to handle. So was his home. So was his split heart.

Sex was where he collapsed. To feel desire these days, he needed to feel that everything was under control: no marital differences, no messy house, no complaining kids, no internal emotional conflict. No wonder he wasn't initiating sex anymore. His conditions were too exacting, and they were never met.

He seemed to understand this idea when we explored it. "But I can't change how I grew up," he said pragmatically. "So what am I to do?"

"One thing you can change," I said, "is your relationship to Ireland."

"You don't want me to give it up, now, do you?" He eyed me suspiciously.

"No," I said. "But if you're going to be internally conflicted about this for the next two or five or twenty years, you need to figure out how to have sexual desire at the same time."

After a moment of silence, the tall redhead spoke. "You're saying I might not fix this California-Ireland problem for a while, then?" This was a new way of looking at it. He had been waiting for the split to magically resolve so he could start his life. "So I have to get on with things now, like making love with my wife?"

"Yes. And while you're at it, learn to appreciate her body as it is, too. It isn't likely to reverse course and magically look ten years younger anytime soon."

He laughed. "Love the one you're with, eh? Doctor, you'd be very popular back in Dublin," he said. "Okay, let's talk about getting hot for my Catherine." So we talked about renewing his attraction to her: seeing her as colorful, not flaky; as a mother who nourished the kids' creativity, not as a poor housekeeper; as a fleshy woman who desired him and was energetic in bed, not as an over-the-hill mum.

And I told him to limit himself to dancing at one wedding per night.

It worked. After only six more sessions, we said good-bye. "Perfection would be great," he said when we parted, "but it's no longer necessary. Enjoying what I have is damn fine," he added with a smile.

Know Your Body as It Is

There are no perfect adult bodies or faces. As supermodel Cindy Crawford used to say, "Even I don't wake up looking like Cindy Crawford."

Your body is, what, a quarter-century old? More? A half-century old? After a few years, everything on earth gets a little beat-up, even our bodies. And things acquire little idiosyncrasies. Your Honda's front tires squeak only when turning left, not right. Your blender leaks at high speeds but not at low speeds. Sometimes it's easier to move your chair than to adjust the overhead light.

If most of the sex you had when young was while you were drunk or stoned, you'll be having sex with a new body now. (Assuming you're not still having sex only when drunk or stoned. You may notice the music has changed since then too.) If you don't have quite the stamina or upper-body strength you had ten years ago, that will also affect your sexual repertoire. In this regard, sex is not sacred—your cardiovascular system thinks it's just another workout, like a stationary bike (without the Kindle or iPod, presumably).

If you began your sexual career with many partners and now you're with only one, your body may respond differently—requiring more warming up, for example. If a lot of your interest in sex has been about conquest and now you're with one regular partner, your body may need new things (positions, games, toys) to get sufficiently excited. And if you've been watching a lot of porn or have become a regular vibrator user, that may affect your body's responses too.

If you now have physical pain in certain positions that didn't bother you before, that's something to admit to yourself and adapt to (that's why there's all those chandeliers for sale on eBay). When familiar activities go from being a source of pleasure to a source of pain, a change is needed—along with the emotional skills to handle the loss. Some people who lack those skills attempt to avoid the necessary change. Denial is one way people end up in the emergency room—whether from choosing ski slopes they can no longer negotiate safely, or from having sex in kama sutra positions that are now far too challenging. Denial is also one way people develop low desire—to avoid acknowledging the physical pain of once-familiar sexual activities.

How Sex Actually Feels in Your Body

Let's take this idea a step further and discuss how your body actually feels during sex. Not how you assume it feels, not what you think about what you're doing, but how things actually feel. The human body brings a huge amount of sensory equipment to every sexual event—much of it unused, misinterpreted, or ignored.

For many of us, attending to our actual experience during sex is more complicated than it sounds. That's because when we keep repeating a certain action or behavior, we eventually do it from habit rather than from a consciousness of being present. That's understandable—if you paid careful attention every time you brushed your teeth or buttoned your shirt, you'd never have time to leave the house, much less actually do anything.

In addition, if you're anxious, you may be so focused on other things that you can't really feel how sex feels. As we've already discussed, during sex people often focus on how they look, sound, or smell; trying to function correctly; trying to ignore physical or emotional pain; or on trying to figure out how their partner is feeling. It's obviously difficult to feel the different parts of your body, and subtle changes in stimulation, when you already have so much on your mind.

Most of us understand this principle in other settings; for example, if you're doing an important job interview in a restaurant, you'll hardly notice how your food tastes. In general, anxiety reduces our ability to experience novel things or to enjoy ourselves.

Here's how that dynamic can work during sex:

- If during sex you're imagining a fantasy in order to get more excited, you'll miss some of the actual sensory experience.

- If you have a judgment about a certain kind of stimulation (fellatio is for whores, nipples are for gay guys, finger-in-vagina is for frigid women or inept men), your prejudice will prevent you from trying it—or actually feeling it if you do.

- If you don't clear your mind before having sex, stray incoming thoughts (chores, work, next week's schedule) can settle there, reducing your focus on your experience.

Perhaps at this point you're asking yourself, "Why should I have to pay attention like this during sex? I didn't have to do that when I was younger."

Yes, that *may* be true. But now you're older, so perhaps you want a fuller, richer (maybe even elegant) experience. And if you've only started having sex sober in the last year or two, your ability to pay attention has increased dramatically. Learning how to do that properly is an art form that has to be mastered; no one is born knowing how to pay attention during sex, and our culture discourages everyone from learning it.

Perhaps you've been watching a sport on TV for years. Some people watch the same way their whole lives; others watch in increasingly complex ways as they understand the game more, over time becoming impatient if confronted with simplistic announcers or a lack of instant replays and multiple cameras. While many people go to Super Bowl parties to drink and talk, others like to stay home and intently watch the game, and they're not complaining about "having" to pay attention to get more enjoyment from watching. They think it's an opportunity for extra pleasure.

It's interesting that people resist paying attention during sex: closing their eyes during sex, too busy creating sex to feel it, afraid of discovering something uncomfortable about themselves, feeling too overwhelmed or alienated by the experience to cuddle afterwards—i.e., to continue the erotic encounter after orgasm, feeling one's body close to another's.

In addition, digital technology and devices like smart phones now encourage a continual splitting of attention that's new and troubling.

Most people assume that multitasking is not only innocent, but advantageous and even necessary to manage the modern world. Research shows that for repetitive tasks like dressing or wiping a kitchen counter, it's a fine way to organize ourselves. For more complex activities, however, not only is multitasking not innocent, it's really detrimental. The first things multitasking undermines are (1) creativity and (2) intimate human connection. Don't you think sex should involve at least one of those? If so, multitasking and sex really don't mix.

American teens send and receive over 3,000 text messages a month, which is one every six minutes that they're not asleep or in school. The rate for kids under twelve is almost half as many messages per month. Adults may say that's crazy—but adults text almost that much. My patients complain about spouses texting at the dinner table; the spouses typically claim they can listen while they text. I think that speaks to the quality of their listening.

Many young people consider it perfectly acceptable to answer their phone or *begin texting* in the middle of a face-to-face conversation with someone. If you're not prepared to say that this custom interferes with human connectedness, let's agree that it changes the meaning of human connectedness. And that certainly changes our internal expectations about intimacy—including sex.

In the 1970s people had to develop an etiquette about using ATMs (for example, how close to the person using it should the first person in line stand?). Similarly, (young) people are right now developing an etiquette about texting after sex: How long afterwards does a polite person wait? How many texts are okay? How much privacy should your sex partner give you while you're texting?

Inevitably, we'll soon see a bunch of romantic comedies in which people are texting *during* sex. If the film *Network* (1976) were remade today, Faye Dunaway would be texting during sex—and William Holden would be confused and dismayed. They were, if you recall, from different generations.

Anyway, you know what Albert Einstein said about multitasking: "Any man who can drive safely while kissing a pretty girl is simply not giving the kiss the attention it deserves."

Redefining "Sexy"

There's an apocryphal story about Don Jose, the most accomplished bullfighter in Spain.

At the height of Don Jose's career, some journalists arrange an interview with him. When they arrive at his spacious home outside Madrid, they find him in the kitchen wearing a frilly apron, washing dishes.

"It's the maid's day off," he explains. "I'm just about finished."

The journalists look at each other, feeling awkward. "Your home is beautiful," they say, "and we appreciate you making the time to see us. But we're confused. You are our national hero, courageous, skillful, the symbol of masculinity to every man and woman in Spain. And here you are wearing a frilly pink apron, so *muy delicado, muy femenino.*"

"Feminine?" he responds, his dark eyes flashing. "Feminine? I am the symbol of masculinity to every man and woman in Spain. Everything I do is manly. If I wear a frilly pink apron, it is manly to do so."

If Don Jose could decide this, so can you. You can decide what is manly, or womanly, or sexy—and you'd be silly to craft a definition that excludes you. It would be like starting a club and writing membership rules in a way that made you ineligible to join.

Why be limited to John Wayne or Kanye West, Mae West or Jessica Alba, *Sex and the City* or *Mad Men* (or *Silence of the Lambs*), or *any* image? We all need to create our own images of what's sexy. Here are a few examples of what you could decide is *muy erotico, muy caliente*:

- Remembering *exactly* how your partner likes her hair touched

- Bringing a special snack to bed

- Kissing with eyes open

- Bringing him socks if his feet are cold

- Taking out the lube as you're getting into bed, instead of waiting until you "need" it

- Gently washing her vulva before sex, or the ejaculate off his chest afterwards

Clinging to overly narrow definitions of ideas like sexy, womanly, "good sex," and "good lover" is a terrible mistake; clinging to definitions that exclude you as you are is not just a mistake, it's the opposite of Sexual Intelligence, a real obstacle to sexual satisfaction. Imagine you're advertising a new car or a new sneaker. Would you apologize to your audience for the product not being perfect, or would you say, *this* is the definition of perfection? Would you say, "I hope you want this," or would you say, "Trust me, *this* is what you've been looking for"?

For people who say, "But such-and-such has been my image of sexiness or masculinity all my life, I can't change it," I say, don't change it then—expand it. Decide that "sexy" can include both Lady Gaga *and* you, that "masculine" is both LeBron James *and* you. You can create any category you want, as long as you personally qualify.

If that sounds too arbitrary, you're half right. It *is* arbitrary—all these categories are. Why Britney Spears one year, Lindsay Lohan the next, and now neither? It's all fads—which means these categories are just arbitrary consensus, with no intrinsic value. In the bedroom, the only consensus necessary is between you and your partner(s). And that starts with you. Decide you're sexy, dammit!

Name one good reason that you refuse.

Communicating to Create Outcomes

In Chapter 5, we talked about the importance of making communication a *technical* skill rather than an *emotional* one. We saw that when someone is afraid of the outcome of communication (whether their reason makes sense or not), he or she naturally hesitates to connect verbally.

And we saw in the last chapter that some people give a special meaning to *not* communicating—that it's romantic, or that it allows sex to be "spontaneous." Not communicating in order to make sex more romantic or spontaneous is like walking barefoot so you don't scuff your shoes. It's like keeping your umbrella in your car so it doesn't get wet in the rain. It's like, as my mother would say, burning down the house to roast the pig.

No, you can get more value from communicating than from not communicating. So let's look at the practical/technical side of communication, starting with a food analogy.

Whether you cook or not, you undoubtedly know hundreds of words for ingredients, kitchen tools, and food preparation. Here are a few examples:

- *Ingredients:* Spices, sauces, vegetables, oils, meats, dairy products, grains, sweeteners, stock

- *Tools and objects:* Pot, strainer, frying pan, measuring cup, bowl, knife, peeler, cutting board, plate, refrigerator, oven, can opener

- *Actions:* Boil, fry, sauté, chop, pour, measure, whisk, mince, steam, mix, toss, slice, bake, stir, nuke (isn't that everyone's word for what a microwave oven does?)

Now imagine a couple trying to cook a meal (or even a snack) together without using words like these. It would sound like this: "Honey, please take the X, and Y it in a Z for a few minutes. Then...."

No matter how good these people are at charades, anything more complicated than pouring a glass of water would be impossible. At best everything would take a really long time. And each person would feel very frustrated. So a common vocabulary is essential whenever two people want to pursue a joint project, from building a birdhouse to throwing a dinner party to cleaning a bathroom to sharing sex. That's why we need words for body parts, erotic activities, and our subjective experience. "Honey, use your y'know to y'know my y'know" doesn't provide much guidance.

Recall the Bible story about the Tower of Babel. When God wanted to stop the construction of a grand edifice that would reach all the way to heaven, God didn't need to take away people's tools or materials. He just had each one suddenly speak a language that no one else could understand. The project screeched to a halt within moments.

A sexual vocabulary is part of Sexual Intelligence, and is absolutely essential for enjoyable sex. If your vocabulary consists primarily of "down there" and "it" and "y'know," it will be hard to guide your partner, inform your partner, or share with your partner. And it's far less likely that you'll get the kind of sexual experiences you want.

So assuming you're convinced that talking about sex with your partner is a great idea, how should you go about it?

Let's start in bed, perhaps during sex.

Dos and Don'ts for Communicating About Sex in Bed

- Ask your partner to do one or more things you know (or you think) you'd like. (Sexually, I mean; this isn't the time to request help installing antivirus software.)

- Talk about what you want more than about what you don't want; for example, instead of saying, "That's too fast," say, "I'd like it slower."

- If you say, "Don't do that," add, "Do this instead."

- Be friendly when talking about sex (unless you're about to climax—in which case demanding something and forgetting to say "please" seems reasonable).

- Unless something dreadful just happened (a condom broke, you discovered your partner's been faking orgasms), save the *serious* conversation for after sex.

- Nothing says, "I'm here with you" like eye contact. Look at your partner periodically during sex, especially when talking or listening. Even "Oh God, oh God!" deserves eye contact, just like "Wait, do that soon but not yet."

- Save "Don't ever do that again" and "How many times do I have to tell you" for after sex is over—either later that day or later that week. Or maybe never.

- Take your partner's hand and stroke yourself (leg, hair, butt, nose, whatever) with it the way you like. Whisper "like this." In fact, whisper a lot. It's sexy.

- Don't talk about how a former partner did something better. Don't talk about how someone else looks better or feels better. Don't talk about how someone else's bed never had cracker crumbs in it.

- Don't ask, "Where did you learn that?" or, "Who taught you to do that?"

- If something feels good, say so.

- If something feels really good, say so more than once.

- Don't ever, ever, ever say that something feels good when it doesn't.

- Don't ask, "Why the hell did you do that?" Just say, "No thanks."

- If your partner says, "I love you," you don't have to say it right back; you can smile, or you can say, "Hmm, good." And never say "I love you" if you don't mean it. Or if you don't plan on saying it again within thirty days.

Sometimes the best time and place to communicate about sex is outside the bedroom. Here are some examples of things to say or discuss when you're *not* in the middle of sex:

Tips for Communicating About Sex in the Kitchen (or Wherever)

- Ask what some word or gesture or face meant.

- Ask what your partner likes, or if he or she likes a certain thing.

- Use the right names for body parts.

- Sit close enough to touch when you talk. Then touch when you talk.

- Discuss and decide on a "safe word"—an unusual word (like *dinosaurs*) that, if either person says it during sex,

means "Stop right now, and I really mean it!" And don't fool
around with the word once you've agreed on it.

- Discuss policy: "Just so you know, I'm not going to want X in
the future, so please don't ask me about it or try it."

- If you aren't sure what your partner meant during the most
recent lovemaking, ask: was that "No, not now," or "No,
not ever"?

- Confirm your contraceptive agreement(s)—what, when,
how? And here's some advice: "trying harder" has no place
in this conversation. Contraception is about what you do,
not about what you try to do, or try to remember to do, or
think you ought to do.

- Clarify and resolve any disagreements about logistics: room
temperature, alcohol during sex, socks in bed, talking nasty,
locking the door, and so on.

- Describe your body's current situation, whether temporary
or permanent: lower back pain, difficulty squeezing your
hands, asthma. If necessary, remind your partner whether
you're right- or left-handed (an important factor when
arranging the bodies for a hand job). Also mention where
you're particularly flexible or strong—for example, hips or
arms (an important resource if someone's getting on their
hands and knees).

- Don't judge what you don't like ("Ugh, that's kinky/perverse/
unromantic"). If you don't want to do something in bed, you
don't need a "good" reason. So you don't have to justify your
lack of interest in it by criticizing the activity or its sponsor.

- Like Amazon.com, you can inquire: "Since you like X (sex-
related act), I wonder if you'd like Y (a slightly similar sex-
related act)."

- "Hey, one of these days when we're in bed together, do you
maybe want to try X?"

- "You should know that when we're not getting along so well, I'm a lot less interested in sex." Unless you're one of the unusual people for whom the truth is, "When we're not getting along, I'm a lot *more* interested in sex."

If you use different words or have different dos and don'ts, but your conversations sound pretty much like these, that's fine—as long as you're communicating with the goals of enhancing clarity and closeness. I know that sometimes over lunch or a drink, a friend tells us a personal story with too many details, and we think, "Um, TMI—that's Too Much Information." But there's almost no such thing in sex—as long as the communication is done with the goals of clarity and closeness, and you're paying attention to what you're doing, more information is almost always better than less information.

Along with paying attention to your conditions, your experiences, and your concepts, communicating is one of the best ways of increasing your Sexual Intelligence.

Chapter Nine

Embracing the Inevitable
Health and Aging Challenges

Kelli was thrilled to get pregnant. As a serious club tennis player, she was already in fantastic shape, so her doctor assured her she'd sail through pregnancy.

A week later she started to puke. And gain weight. And hate everyone.

Her husband, Hector, dutifully backed off their regular sex schedule (usually about twice per week), telling himself it was only temporary and that she obviously felt wretched. Besides, she didn't seem like she'd be much fun to play with right now.

After three months, Kelli's hormones calmed down and she stopped puking. As her belly got rounder, she gradually seemed like her old self, and resumed being nice to everyone—except her husband. In particular, she didn't want to have sex with him. She didn't even want to kiss him, saying his breath made her nauseous.

Unlike some other husbands who tease, embarrass, or reject their pregnant wives, Hector was still affectionate, regularly telling Kelli how attractive she was and how he desired her.

Meanwhile, she was getting bigger and bigger, and she didn't like it one bit.

At first she had various reasons for her withdrawal from Hector, then excuses, and in their first big blowup about it, she accused her husband of being insincere about finding her attractive in her current state. Stunned, he told her how beautiful she was. "You're just desperate to get laid after all these months," she scolded. When he denied this, she just got angrier. After weeks and weeks of this recurring battle, she said, during a session, "He doesn't really want me, he's just trying to make me feel better. Well, I can see right through him, and it's not working. I'm not an idiot—I know I look like a damn whale."

Kelli claimed she could live with Hector being honest and rejecting her while pregnant, but she couldn't stand what she perceived as his dishonesty, "obviously" patronizing and manipulating her.

Hector was baffled and hurt, and after trying to connect with her for months, he withdrew. The situation was looking worse and worse. I also had my eye on the calendar: in just eleven weeks Kelli would give birth, and their lives would really be turned upside down. That would be no time to put the marriage back together; I really wanted to do it now, accomplishing as much as possible before she gave birth. In some ways I had a stronger sense of urgency than they did, never a good setup for therapy.

How could I get Kelli to consider the possibility that Hector was telling the truth, and that she was actually expressing her own disgust about herself? "Kelli, what if he's telling the truth?" I asked. "Then," she replied angrily, "either he doesn't care how I look anymore, which sucks, or he never really saw or cared about how I looked before, which sucks, or I'm making this whole thing up and I'm crazy. I don't know which is worse."

The first two were completely false.

Truly, she was projecting her self-rejection onto him. For years she had been highly identified with her body—not so much her looks, but her mobility, gracefulness, and feline trimness. She had lost these—and was afraid she'd never get them back. She'd think about it, feel selfish for thinking about it, wonder if getting pregnant had been such a good idea, and then start the cycle again.

One week, out of nowhere, she asked, "Is it safe to have sex while I'm pregnant?" It turned out she was also afraid that she'd lose her sexuality, another thing with which she was strongly identified. I asked what her doctor had said. "Oh, she said it was okay, but I don't know if I believe her. She doesn't look like she's ever had sex, and Hector and I can get, well, you know, we're both kind of athletic. . . ." He laughed, and she smiled shyly. It was sweet.

"Not only can you have sex now," I said, "you can also have sex after you give birth."

"But I hear it takes a year or two before couples have sex again," she said. "I don't like that. And how is Hector going to manage?"

I assured her that if it took a year, it took a year; they'd be fine. (I felt this was ultimately more instructive than assuring her that it probably wouldn't take nearly that long.) Hector made a few jokes, all with the theme of "I'll wait for you."

Not only was Kelli concerned about Hector being turned off to her body now; she was concerned that either her body would be "permanently disfigured" and he'd be turned off forever, or that she'd lose weight and regain her old body, but he'd then be turned off by the ugly picture of her that would supposedly be seared into his memory.

"You don't get it," the usually calm husband finally said one day. "And I'm tired of it." Hector hardly ever talked that way. "You seem to have a problem with your looks now, and you seem to be afraid that I'll think you're ugly for the rest of our lives. That's ridiculous," he said. "You insist you can predict exactly how I'll feel, but you're wrong."

"If necessary," he continued, "we can go without sex the rest of your pregnancy. That will be lousy, but I can manage it. But we are going to have sex after the baby comes, and it will be just as great as it used to be. Right?" She was impassive. "Right? Right?" He turned to me in frustration.

"It's never going to be like it was," she finally said in a voice of quiet desperation. "You'll be the same sexy guy, so of course I'll eventually desire you again. So will other women. But I'm ruined forever. You won't want me, I'm already disgusted with myself, and nobody but losers will think I'm attractive."

"You're absolutely right," I told Kelli, to Hector's surprise. "It's never going to be like it was. The question is, can you two make it wonderful in a new way? Kelli, you seem to believe your husband's sexual interest in you is pretty shallow; with that belief, of course you're anxious about the future. If you listen, maybe you'll learn something about Hector."

Indeed, Kelli had never stopped worrying long enough to realize that Hector desired her for more than her perfect body. "Kelli, I want you to imagine that there's more than one way Hector can desire you and see you as attractive, more than one way that people can connect sexually. Once you do that," I said, "everything else is just details. When you insist that Hector is terribly inflexible in his desire for his wife, you're saying more about your imagination than about his.

"Fortunately," I continued, "Hector will bring his imagination and his desire for you to your marriage no matter how skeptical or self-conscious you are. His desire for you is like gravity—even if you don't believe in it, it's still real. It would be a real waste to insist that Hector doesn't desire you when he does."

"You're asking me to trust him an awful lot," Kelli said slowly. I agreed. She said she wasn't sure she could do that just now.

"Yes, maybe it isn't something you want to do now."

Kelli noticed my reframe. "You make it sound like a choice," she said.

Again I nodded: "Yes, I believe it starts as a decision to trust, and then we figure out how to do it."

Kelli didn't quite agree, but she noticed that it could give her a way out of her dilemma. That was good enough for me—until our next session, anyway.

✳ ✳ ✳

Most of us develop our model of sexuality when we have the body of a young, healthy person. Most of us only have that body for a few years, and no one has it more than a decade or two. So if we want to enjoy sex when we develop a different body, we better have a different model of sexuality available.

Without that vision, we will have difficulty sustaining our desire, as we will question our attractiveness and our very eligibility for sexiness. If our partner is close to our age, we'll have a hard time seeing him or her as attractive or desirable too.

Aging and health issues have tremendous effects on people's sexual experience. Matters of concern include medication side effects; sex during pregnancy and after childbirth; sexual effects of contraception; reduced stamina or range of motion; menopause; chronic pain; and unwanted changes in the body's functions, including desire, lubrication, erection, and orgasm.

Using the standards of what a young person's body can do during sex (stamina, flexibility, desire, erection, lubrication, orgasm, and so on), many people over thirty-five will "fail" at sex over and over. Rather than enjoying what an older body and an older mind can create during sex, too many people focus on comparing who they *are* with who they *were*. This is terribly distracting, whether we like the comparison or not.

To enhance sexual satisfaction past age thirty-five, you need to come to terms with this new context for sex. After all, "good sex" for you will never again look like it's "supposed to"—if that requires two young, healthy bodies. Especially if you (or your partner) have one or more common health challenges, you need to feel empowered to redefine "sexy" to include someone—yourself—in a physical state that society specifically defines as *unsexy*.

Only then can you take advantage of facts and techniques that can make sex more enjoyable. Otherwise, it's like taking piano lessons while listening to an iPod. Even the best teaching in the world won't get through.

As we've already seen, it's important to establish your own idiosyncratic model of sexuality—enjoying what you choose to put in, and grieving what you've lost and therefore can't put in. There's so much (faux) cheerfulness in the media about "successful aging" and "lifelong sexual vitality" that I think many people underestimate the emotional difficulties. It's like a travel brochure for Cuba that features the beautiful beaches, the great music, and the gorgeous women but doesn't mention the grinding poverty.

Common Health Problems
with Sexual Impacts

You'll recall our discussion of "erogenous zones"—how it's a limited concept, and how the entire body can be the site of sexual feelings.

I believe the concept of sexual "function" and "dysfunction" is similarly limited, because it makes an artificial distinction between bodily reactions that are sexual and those that aren't. A blinding migraine that turns a romantic weekend into a lonely nightmare is just as much a sexual problem as an unreliable erection or a burning feeling in your vagina.

So before we get into some specifics about health and aging challenges, let's note some of the "non-sexual" health problems that often have sexual consequences:

☐ Insomnia	☐ Irritable bowel syndrome
☐ Diabetes	☐ Asperger's syndrome
☐ Arthritis	☐ Obesity
☐ Chronic fatigue syndrome	☐ Hormone disorders
☐ Fibromyalgia	☐ Tinnitus
☐ Asthma	☐ Carpal tunnel syndrome
☐ Migraines	☐ Depression
☐ Hypertension	☐ Dementia
☐ Degenerative disk disease	☐ Sciatica
☐ Yeast and urinary infections	☐ Hypothyroidism
☐ Lupus	☐ Sjogren's syndrome

. . . and anything else that makes it hard for people to get along, be nice to each other, spend time together, pay attention, or enjoy their bodies.

If you're thinking, "Wow, it seems like practically every illness has a sexual component"—yes, I think that's accurate.

_____

People experience health challenges at all ages, so facing one doesn't make you "old." That said, many of the insights and strategies we'll be discussing here apply in similar ways to the challenges posed to sex by aging.

You've already read about a range of Sexual Intelligence tools that will help you understand and approach the sexual challenges of health and aging. These include:

- Talking with your mate

- Letting go of sexual hierarchies

- Realizing that you give sex meaning rather than sex having inherent meaning

- Deciding what your conditions for good sex are and communicating these to your partner

- Letting go of the need for "spontaneity" in sex

Now let's discuss how to apply these tools and ideas.

Sexual Effects of Medications

Many prescription drugs have sexual side effects, which can undermine desire, slow down arousal, and inhibit orgasm. Some common drugs with sexual side effects are:

- Antidepressants
- Diuretics (used for hypertension)
- Analgesics (pain medication)
- Antihistamines
- Anti-anxiolytics (used for anxiety)
- Anti-epileptics
- Antihypertensives
- Appetite suppressants
- Oral contraceptives
- Cancer chemotherapy

Medications don't have to affect sexual function directly in order to impact your sexual experience or sexual relationships. Some medications affect sexuality in other ways:

- Making your mouth taste funny
- Making you thirsty all the time
- Making you sleepy
- Making you mentally sluggish
- Making you grind your teeth, snore, or shake
- Requiring you to not drink alcohol
- Changing the smell of your sweat or breath
- Making you prone to depression

Effects like these can inhibit kissing and oral sex, make you less attractive as a partner, alienate you from your own body or sexuality, or simply make sex a lower priority in your life.

Not surprisingly, the sexual side effects of drugs are one of the main reasons people don't comply with their doctor's orders about how frequently and for how long to take a medicine. (If that sounds like you, make an appointment with your doctor this week to review and possibly change your drug regimen.)

Unfortunately, many doctors don't discuss this with patients when prescribing a new drug. The same is true with the pharmacists who dispense them. These professionals should know how common sexual side effects are, and how these side effects often discourage patients from taking their medicine. Doctors and pharmacists should take the initiative to discuss sexual side effects with patients. Unfortunately, shyness, lack of information, fear of the patient's response, and a misplaced sense of courtesy or propriety often get in their way.

If you do have sexual difficulties while taking medication, you can:

- Talk with your pharmacist

- Talk with your physician

- Talk with your therapist

- Talk with your partner

Also, ask yourself: did my sexual difficulties begin or get worse when I started the medication? Sometimes we feel so glad about the positive impact of a drug that we don't realize the drug might also be contributing negatively to our lives.

While we're on the subject, let's briefly look at recreational drugs. The common ones—marijuana, cocaine, and the amphetamine family—have an interesting effect on sexuality. Most users say that a little bit makes them more interested in sex, while a lot makes them less interested. So while moderation may not be the key to happiness in all things, it does increase the chances that you can enjoy sex when you're using a street drug.

How Many Street Drugs Affect Sexual Response

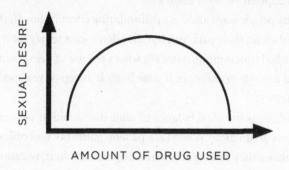

Effects of Alcohol on Sexuality
===============================

Effects of Alcohol on Sexuality

Alcohol is a drug too, and it has well-known effects on the human mind and body.

For thousands of years, people have described alcohol as a drug that disinhibits; i.e., it makes people feel more relaxed, less anxious, less embarrassed, more willing to take chances, less concerned with social convention. Thus, it allows people to do things they wouldn't ordinarily do, or wouldn't do without discomfort.

At the same time, alcohol reduces the speed of people's reflexes, reduces hand-eye coordination, inhibits motor discrimination, slurs their speech, and ultimately makes them sleepy. Thus, it makes subtle physical gestures more difficult or even impossible. That's why both bras and condom packages become harder to open. Alcohol also makes it harder to get or keep an erection and interferes with vaginal lubrication.

So there's the conflict, which Shakespeare described so well in *Macbeth*: alcohol "provokes the desire, but takes away the performance." And so "lechery, sir, it provokes *and* unprovokes." That is, it reduces our inhibitions—which many people want regarding sex—but it makes it harder to "perform"—to allow or make our bodies do what we want them to.

Many people want alcohol's disinhibiting effect (if not on themselves, then on their partner), but they don't want to pay for it with diminished functioning. After all, what's the use of being mentally relaxed enough to enjoy sex if your body is asleep or you can't feel your limbs?

So where is the ideal balance of *some* disinhibition without *too much* loss of function? When I ask patients, students, and colleagues to estimate, they often guess three drinks, even four, occasionally five. (Anyone seriously guessing five has either never had a drink, or is incredibly anxious about sex.) While it's different for each person, the answer for most people is actually about one drink. That's right—for most people, after only two-thirds of a drink, more alcohol actually degrades the sexual experience by removing more in function than it adds in relaxation and playfulness.

How Alcohol Affects Sexual "Function"

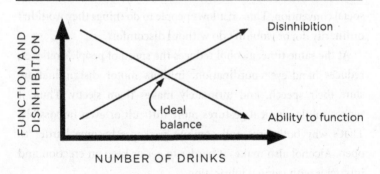

Now, after about one drink, most people believe that more alcohol *doesn't* cost them much in functioning—because as we drink we're typically getting less and less sensitive to what our body is doing and feeling. And because when we're drunk, almost anything that doesn't make us angry can seem funny. At the time. You know, "You had to be there."

So alcohol is another drug that, when it comes to sex—moderation is best.

A Special Note About Chronic Pain

Chronic pain: it's aggravating, tiring, embarrassing, and it's a life sentence.

People who have it get tired of talking about it; people who don't have it get tired of hearing about it. Meanwhile, it's the silent third party in the bedroom. Sex involves Ron, George, and Ron's pain.

It's such a betrayal. Almost everyone with chronic pain remembers when they didn't have it: "Oh, *those* were the days!"

No one wants to adjust their lovemaking to chronic pain. It makes someone feel old, weak, vulnerable, self-conscious, not-sexy. Pathetic. And it forces a person to accept the finality of the pain, the fact that it isn't a temporary problem—it's a permanent one. That alone is why so many people don't adapt their lovemaking to their pain—the increase in pleasure simply isn't worth the depressing reminder of the horrifying truth. No, better for sex to hurt than for sex to be a reminder that this pain is permanent. Better to lose interest in sex than for sex to be a reminder that this pain is permanent.

If you know (or suspect) that your partner hurts during sex, grab him or her, snatch away the Snickers or the TV remote, and tell your partner, "You're busted!" You're from the Pain Squad, and you insist that the two of you talk; specifically, how exactly can the two of you adapt your sex so it hurts less? (See, we're going for less pain rather than no pain—how awful is that already?)

Adapting to reduce pain might be as simple as switching sides of the bed, or switching positions, or using pillows under the butt, shoulder, ankles, or neck. Or it may involve taking ibuprofen or a hot bath a few minutes before sex. Or it may involve a five-minute massage—neck, shoulders, hands, whatever—right before sex, or three minutes of lying quietly and breathing, relaxing the body and visualizing comfortable muscles and joints right before sex. People rarely do that without being pushed. So push. Oh, and then help pick up the pieces of your partner's existential crisis that results from acknowledging that he or she is living with chronic pain.

Damaged Body Image

In America, we learn to feel ashamed when our body's outside doesn't match who we feel we are on the inside. That's true for the signs of aging (such as wrinkles), as well as for a wide range of other body features: weight, posture, facial asymmetry, fitness, scars, visible injury, and artificial devices (braces, cane, wheelchair, and so on). All these issues can create a contrast between the way we look to others (and, especially, in the mirror) and the healthy, "normal" way we feel on the inside.

We can all understand this. I know I don't *feel* like a person my age and my weight—but when you look at me, that's exactly what you see, and of course you assume that what you see is accurate. That's one reason many people get upset about their bodies—the body is the vehicle through which, we assume, others are misjudging who we are.

This is a pretty routine, if painful, part of adolescence (a dangerous one for some), but for many people it starts again (or continues) when they reach their thirties, or after childbirth, when they go bald, when they retire, and at many other times. It's a common complaint: "How could I look this way? I feel sexy (or young), but my body doesn't look it (at least not to me)."

So our distress is about one, two, or all three of these things: the beauty thing (I don't look as good as I want to or used to); the dissonance thing (how I look doesn't reflect who I feel I am); and the definition-of-sexy thing (I know I don't fit the official definition of sexy, but trust me, I am).

Both aging and illness demand that a person problematize his or her body. Ordinarily, adults wrestling with aging or a disease relate to their troublesome body mostly by (grudgingly) taking care of it and (resentfully) working around it. When your body is the focus of so much frustration, disappointment, sadness, and powerlessness, it can be hard to imagine your body as a focus of your pleasure and of others' desire and delight.

And so you have to remember that being sexy is about who you are, not how you appear. As someone gets to know and appreciate you, your body comes along for the ride. You should treat your body like an honored guest, not an albatross.

Of course, this is all especially true when you're in the bedroom and your clothes come off. You feel self-conscious. You're afraid your partner will be disappointed, perhaps imagining how you looked ten or twenty years ago. If you're uncomfortable with your body's appearance, you must, must, must ignore how the damn thing looks and allow sex to happen, uninterrupted by your self-consciousness or judgments. Our culture, of course, is not your ally in this; as sexual anthropologist Mickey Diamond says, "Nature loves diversity. Unfortunately, society hates it."

What You Can Expect with Aging

Let's look at some of the common changes you may experience while you age, and compare these with some things about your sexuality that may *not* change as you get older. What do I mean by "aging" and "older"? Some vague time around forty. But your mileage may vary substantially. Some people are sexually exhausted by thirty, while some late bloomers are just getting started in middle age.

First, what are common *changes* in sexuality with aging?

- *Desire:* Often declines.

- *Vaginal lubrication:* Typically declines in volume and consistency.

- *Erection:* Requires more stimulation; may not be as hard or last as long.

- *Orgasm:* May take longer to arrive; may not last as long or be as powerful.

- *Refractory period:* The mandatory waiting time between ejaculation and next erection often increases.

- *Preferences:* The typical sexual repertoire may shrink; experimentation often declines. Occasionally it works in reverse: some people who have been inhibited for twenty or thirty years get a new lease on life (new partner? near-death experience? Mom remarries?), and their sexual menu expands as they become more experimental.

Second, how can sexuality *remain stable* with aging? Whether the following aspects of sexuality start low in youth and stay low throughout adulthood, or start high in youth and stay high in adulthood, they can remain stable over time:

- Desire for closeness

- Desire to be desired

- Desire to feel good in your own body

- Experience of orgasm

- Level of desire

- Content and quantity of fantasy

- Preferences

Sexual "Function" and Age: Some Changes, Some Constants

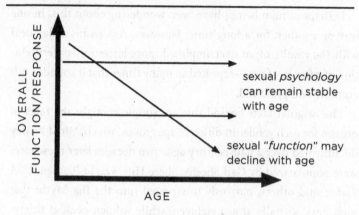

So note that while sexual *function* often changes with age, sexual *psychology* can remain stable over time. Sexual Intelligence gives you the tools and motivation to shift your sexuality as you get older to accommodate this contrast. That's one important way in which you can continue to enjoy sex as your body's ability to do what it used to do declines.

So aging isn't some thief that steals your sexuality; it steals one *version* of your sexuality—function-based sexuality. When it does, you get to decide whether or not your sexuality has left you altogether. If you have emotional courage and sufficient interest, you can reinvent yourself sexually, constructing a satisfying sex life from the familiar pieces of your psychology, using it to work around the changes in your function.

The Myth of Reaching Our "Sexual Peak"

A lot of people are concerned about when they're going to reach their "sexual peak." Will it be high enough? Will it be at the right time? How will it fit with their partner's "sexual peak"? When it comes to sex, America seems filled with mountain climbers.

Perhaps human beings have been wondering about this, in one way or another, for a long time. However, Americans today deal with the results of an oversimplified, popularized misinterpretation of a few key facts—repeated so many times that it sounds both accurate and profound.

The original facts behind this are simple enough: the rates of orgasm for each gender in different age groups, which Alfred Kinsey documented over a half-century ago. Two decades later these rates were popularized by Gail Sheehy, Shere Hite, David Reuben, *USA Today*, and others, narrowly interpreted into the Big Myth: that men peak sexually at age eighteen, while women peak at thirty-five. If that were true, things would be a little messy, but it would hardly be the end of the world. Unfortunately, people have worried about this ever since.

Reasonable answers to the question "when do I reach my sexual peak?" include:

- The question makes no sense.

- I know you're concerned, but the question makes no sense.

- People never reach their sexual peak.

- It depends on what you mean.

If by "sexual peak" you mean quickness to, and hardness of, erection; and if you mean rapidity and propulsive force of ejaculation; and if you mean constantly thinking about and making dumbass jokes about sex; then, yes, many men peak around eighteen. And if by "sexual peak" you mean the age at which women are more sexually responsive and more reliably orgasmic, then, yes, many women peak around thirty-five.

But this pair of definitions is only one way to understand "sexual peak." For example, "sexual peak" could mean the age at which people enjoy sex the most, value it the most, understand it the most, have the most experience, or use it to connect emotionally with their partner the most.

"Sexual peak" could mean the age at which people have the most spiritual experiences with sex, or find it the most psychologically comforting in the face of sorrow, pain, or fear. At the other end of the spectrum, "sexual peak" could mean the age at which some people could most easily sell their sexual services. So if we're going to use the expression "sexual peak" (which I am certainly *not* encouraging), we need to define it as thoughtfully as possible, respecting our own experience and aspirations.

Let's look at the same question in another context: sports in which people run and chase a ball, such as tennis, basketball, baseball, and football.

Virtually everyone playing these sports professionally starts playing by age fourteen. While their youthful bodies can be incredibly fit, they haven't learned much about the game or competition by fourteen, and so there's a limit to how well even these blindingly talented future professional athletes can play.

At twenty-four, professionals can play these sports at incredibly high levels—their bodies are fit and their knowledge is accumulating, especially if they're well coached. At thirty-four, most athletes' bodies have already slowed down a step—but because of their incredible experience and insight into the sport and their opponents, they can still compete at a very high level, even making their teammates better at the same time. Beyond forty-four, all the knowledge in the world can't compensate for the slower feet, slower hands, slower eyes, or slower reactions. We almost never see someone play ball professionally at that age.

For some people, performance is so important that their skill level defines how much they can enjoy a sport. But many people find other things in sports that can be important as well—sometimes even more so. For example:

- The thrill of competition
- The familiarity of the game
- The camaraderie of teammates
- The fresh air
- Wearing the special clothes or uniform
- The sense of mastering the science and strategy of the game
- Hanging out with younger players

If you ask people who love to play sports when they're forty or fifty or even older, most say the same thing: "It isn't like it used to be." Some wish it could be, while others enjoy it even better now. But they all agree, "I really like it the way it is." In one way, they've all passed their peak as players. On the other hand, if they still enjoy playing way longer than they thought they would, and long after most of their peers have retired, who's to say they've passed their peak?

So when do men and women reach their "sexual peak"? For people no longer interested in sex, they already did. For those still interested in sex, they haven't yet. And if they're fortunate, they never will.

Talking to and Teaching Your Doctor About Sex (and Your Body)

You'd be shocked to discover how little doctors learn about sex in medical school. It's the only thing they do less than sleep.

The attitude at most medical schools is: "Let's teach these people about important stuff, like things that will kill you (or really exotic diseases we have a big grant to study)." So your gynecologist probably knows ten times as much about cervical cancer as about sexual function. If you have cervical cancer, that's a good thing; if not, your doctor may have trouble providing the care you actually need.

Many doctors have told me they're concerned that if they bring up sexual topics, the patient will be offended. I generally say, "Tell them this is the high standard of care in your office, and let them be offended." I walk this walk myself; many of my new patients are offended at my seemingly impertinent questions about sex, and my use of straightforward language to ask these questions. After a while, they generally understand my focus. Some still don't like it, but at least they understand. I remember one patient who used to say exasperatedly, "Can't you call it 'down there' like everyone else?"

In contrast, when I encourage my patients to raise sex questions with their doctors, they typically say, "Oh, my doctor would die of embarrassment if I brought up sex." So like a bunch of nervous drivers at a four-way stop sign, everyone's waiting for the other one to go first. You could be sitting at 6th & Main for hours.

Let's also remember who mostly goes to medical school—people barely old enough to vote. Personally, I'm not entirely comfortable handing my prostate over to a guy who spent his Wonder Years in a library instead of learning about life; on the other hand, it beats the alternative—a doc who *didn't* spend years and years in the medical school library.

I once taught sexuality to medical students at Stanford University. They were bright, earnest, and altogether the least sexually knowledgeable group of twenty-three-year-olds I'd ever met. If you're fortunate, one of these brilliant people is now your doctor.

The moral of the story: just as you have to train your doctor about the idiosyncrasies of your skin (you burn even when it rains), your breasts (lumpy your whole life), and the rest of your body, you have to teach him or her to talk about sex with you: the sexual side effects of drugs, the contraceptive effectiveness of withdrawal, how irregular periods affect your life, questions about the safety of anal sex, why your nipples leak a bit even though you're not pregnant, how to masturbate when you have arthritis, allergies to sperm or latex, the fact that your husband isn't your main sex partner.

Let the docs deal with their discomfort. They're getting paid, and it'll benefit their personal lives.

A Personal Story

Some years ago, I injured my hand pretty badly and spent months in physical therapy. A few members of the staff were intrigued by my work, and I got to know them a little bit. To show my appreciation, one day I offered to give a lecture in the hospital. As it turned out, they were hosting an upcoming regional conference for hand injury professionals (physical and occupational therapists, sports trainers, and so on), and a speaker had just canceled. I arranged to fill in, with the topic "Sexual Issues in Hand Injuries."

As we agreed, about a month later I showed up at the auditorium where the conference was being held. After being introduced, I looked at the two hundred people there, thanked them for the invitation, and asked, "Have you ever noticed how cranky hand injury patients are?" I got the strong positive reaction you might expect—laughing, complaining, head-shaking, swearing, people making jokes.

"Okay," I continued, "I know you talk to these patients about everything—adapting their kitchens, their bathrooms, driving, lifting their babies. So how many of you talk to your hand injury patients about masturbation?"

It was suddenly as quiet as a country road at midnight. "Well," I concluded, "why do you think they're so cranky? They have trouble masturbating—some of them can't do it for months!" Most of the group laughed and laughed; when the surprised laughter subsided, replaced by rueful recognition, I smiled. "Let's talk about the best way to discuss sex with your patients, and why you may have overlooked the importance of the topic."

I think a few old-timers are still talking about that presentation.

Myths About Health and Aging

Despite the enormous amount of accurate information out there and our increased access to it, there are still too many prejudices and wrong ideas circulating as fact.

So let's end with a quiz on Myths About Sexuality, Health, and Aging.

True or False?

(Answers appear on page 204.)

- Older women generally don't climax when they have sex.

- Like younger men, older men need to climax to feel sexually satisfied.

- On the whole, older people aren't sexual.

- Birth control pills frequently lead to cancer.

- Abortion frequently leads to depression.

- Most men who lose desire for their wives or girlfriends are deficient in testosterone.

- If you aren't pregnant after five months of trying, you or your partner is infertile.

- Men mostly like big breasts; without them, a woman shouldn't expect much desire from her mate.

- Most people are more sexually sophisticated when they drink.

- If a man can't get erect, he can't really enjoy sex.

- You can't get pregnant the first time you have sex, or standing up, or if you douche right away.

- If a woman can't climax from intercourse alone, sex therapy, medication, or a new partner will probably make it possible.

- Every year many older guys drop dead from too-vigorous sex—often with prostitutes or during affairs.

- Sex after the first three months of pregnancy is generally unwise.

- Most doctors know everything about sex they need to know.

- Most medications have few or no sexual side effects.

- Good-looking people are the best lovers and have the best sex.

- Erection drugs like Viagra work great for women.

- Almost all sexual "dysfunctions" can be traced to trauma, such as rape, molestation, or childhood deprivation.

- Erection problems are, of course, almost always primarily about sex.

- If you have a sexually transmitted infection (such as herpes or chlamydia), no one will want to have intercourse with you—and it's irresponsible to even suggest it.

Answers to quiz:
All of these statements are false.
There's nothing "controversial" about any of them.
Some people may have feelings about the facts,
but the facts are beyond question.

Regardless of gender, race, political views, or ability to make risotto, "getting older" is the one category that everyone is heading toward. (It beats the alternative, right?) For most people, aging will bring special challenges to expressing sexuality joyfully. For those who already struggle with health problems—because of pain, medication, insomnia, or disease—those challenges to meaningful sexual expression are already here.

It's hard enough losing our cherished sources of pleasure, whether they involve food, sports, child-rearing, traveling, or sex. As we get older or struggle with health problems, it is essential that we use our Sexual Intelligence to reimagine and reinvent sex. That is how we can continue to use sexuality as a source of nourishment, rather than losing it to a narrow set of rigid definitions that inevitably exclude us.

As we have seen, however, some people are so angry or frightened about the necessity of changing their sexual vision that they refuse to do it. They gain the benefits of denial, but they pay for it in their lost sexuality. I can't honestly say this is a mistake for everyone—only that it's a mistake for most people. As the philosophers tell us, pain is mandatory—but suffering is optional.

Chapter Ten

Creating Sex That Can't
Fail (or Succeed)
Using Your Sexual Intelligence

McCoy and Crystal were a nice couple in their mid-thirties. A bit more traditional than many of my patients, they were Russian Orthodox, each with family in the area. They had a child and really wanted another—but before they conceived again, they agreed, they had to work out their "intimate life." They wanted sex that had more "energy" and "closeness," with less "stress" and less arguing.

They were not just inhibited, they were constricted. They thought they knew what sex was supposed to be like, and since they more or less agreed on how that looked, they didn't question their vision. That job fell to me.

We talked about their relationship, which was fairly traditional: he was the main breadwinner, while she was a part-time nurse who raised their child and took care of their home. We discussed issues like power, autonomy, and disagreements. And we discussed their image of their church.

McCoy wasn't that engaged in it; Crystal went to church most weeks, although she said that things like birth control and sex were "personal" issues they decided for themselves. I noted this sense of independence, assuming it would come in handy later.

It was interesting discussing sex with them. As we talked about various practicalities, they took turns not wanting to change. McCoy, for example, hated using a lubricant during sex—he felt they shouldn't "have to," that it meant there was something wrong with Crystal's arousal. She felt that sex had to include intercourse—that "men really need it."

He didn't like the idea of oral sex—he said that it was what prostitutes did for men, and that a "real man" wouldn't go down on a woman. She didn't want to make dates for sex, because she felt they should come together "spontaneously," or else it was "too mechanical, not romantic." And she only wanted to use the so-called missionary position for intercourse, because some others "weren't ladylike," while still others "put too much attention on my backside or breasts, which aren't exactly perfect."

Unintentionally, they were skillfully cooperating to stay stuck. Their ideas about sex undermined the possibility of sexual intimacy. Working so hard to do sex right and make it successful, they couldn't just relax and enjoy each other in bed.

"Well, there's good news," I said cheerily. "You have plenty of reasons that sex isn't the way you want it. There are plenty of things here to change."

I explained how these judgments, interpretations, labels, and so on got in the way of intimacy, which was what they said they wanted. "Putting two naked bodies together for sex, that isn't hard," I said. "Putting them together when you're in a playful mood, or getting in a playful mood when you've put the nude bodies together, that's a little harder.

"You've asked for sex to be more intimate, which is great," I said. "But how exactly do you intend to create that? It isn't a matter of special positions or toys or tricks. It's a matter of getting and staying connected intimately while you happen to be having sex."

I helped them see that each was avoiding the other during sex, didn't really trust they'd be accepted by the other, and wanted an intimate experience without acting in an intimate way. They didn't want to admit that, fearing it meant they didn't love each other; I assured them that wasn't what it "meant."

Sex isn't "intimate" just because it's sex; you have to do stuff to make it intimate. Sometimes people don't realize they have to; sometimes people don't realize they aren't. Sometimes people think it's their partner's responsibility, either because of gender or more experience or tradition or shame.

This couple thought they were doing something wrong because the sex didn't feel "intimate." "Of course it doesn't," I smiled. "You're not relaxing and shaping the sex the way, say, you shape a picnic with your kid. Why aren't you tense then?"

"Because we know what to do," McCoy said.

"I think you do, but I don't think that's why you're relaxed about it. I think it's because you don't worry about doing it right, you're not trying to follow a script, and you don't worry that if things go awry it will be a terrible mess." They nodded thoughtfully. "Now take that same mind-set into sex, and I believe you'll be able to relax and make it intimate."

In just five sessions, that's what happened. McCoy and Crystal started seeing what they were doing, started doing it less, and started talking about how they were perpetuating their own problems. I suggested a few things and encouraged them to leave therapy with me (even though I enjoyed working with them). They added some things to their sexual routine: more kissing, more oral sex, two new positions. They still resisted what they felt was my "attack on intercourse," and McCoy was still tense about Crystal climaxing so much more easily with a vibrator than with him.

But in the end, we demystified sex. It became more real to them—something they needed to shape and manage, not just wait around for, hoping it would be intimate, while passively accepting whatever they got.

✳ ✳ ✳

The Sexual Intelligence model we've been exploring together is a concept of sex that makes it impossible for you to "fail" because you're not aiming for "success." Without measuring yourself against some standard of "normal," you have only two standards left: "How do I like it?" and "Does my partner enjoy this with me?" Since there's nothing to succeed at, you don't have to wait until the sex is over to decide how it was. Instead, you can enjoy virtually every moment along the way, since you already know how the sex ends—it ends with everything being fine. Not perfect perhaps, but fine.

In this vision of sex, nothing can go wrong because there is no "wrong" and no "right." Lost erections, quick climaxes, dry vaginas—they're all just features of sex, not an interruption or a failure. In this erotic world, there's no cultural hierarchy stating that certain kinds of sex are better than others; thus, whatever (consensual) activities people do are fine. Those old hierarchies (intercourse is better than oral sex, oral sex is better than a hand job, toes are inherently not sexy, and so on) are for accountants, not lovers. Unless you want to conceive, they're completely arbitrary, and best ignored.

Ultimately, the Sexual Intelligence approach results in you owning sex, rather than serving it; you end up being free to create (and enjoy) sex, rather than being enslaved by the need to fulfill a cultural model of sexual adequacy. And that's better than any orgasm could possibly be.

———————

In Chapter 1, I promised we would envision and create sex as a place where mistakes are simply not possible, and virtually nothing can go wrong.

I hope you've done that along with me, as we've discussed practical ideas and strategies including:

- Pursuing what you say you want from sex;

- Eliminating your performance orientation, making sex a place to relax instead of a place to succeed (or fail);

- Abandoning the question of whether you or your partner are sexually normal;

- The importance of communicating about sex—and how to do it effectively;

- Realistic sexual physiology: accepting that arousal can fluctuate, sexual response often changes with age, and emotions affect the way your body responds before and during sex;

- The importance of bodily attunement before and during sex, and the value of slowing down to help facilitate it;

- The mistake of identifying certain body parts as "erogenous zones";

- The importance of preparing for and coming to terms with the fact that sex may be different as you move forward in life, so you can enjoy it;

- The importance of focusing on sexual enjoyment rather than sexual function.

Indeed, recall that in all of our discussions, sexual "function"—erection, lubrication, orgasm—is seen as a means to create experiences you desire, rather than an end in itself.

———————

You'll recall that I started this book by asking what people want from sex. Most adults—including, presumably, you—emphasize some kind of closeness or intimacy. So here are some questions I ask patients to help them think about this issue:

- If intimacy is such a big part of sex, why not discuss sex with your mate? Or why tolerate your mate's silence about it?

- If sex is at least partly about intimacy, and you can't or won't communicate, how do you expect to build the intimacy that nourishes enjoyable sex?

- How do you expect to talk about sex if you don't have the words you need?

- How do you expect to make sex intimate or close if you emotionally hide during it?

Although I do it as gently as I can, my patients squirm when I ask questions like these, and if you're squirming a bit now too, I'm very sympathetic. Still, if closeness and intimacy are important parts of sex for you, you need to behave in ways that lead to closeness and intimacy. I've been talking about practical ways to do this throughout the book; below are some additional ideas for creating closeness during sex by making sex a place in which you can't fail. That's the ultimate in Sexual Intelligence.

Don't start sex before you feel close—or ready.

While you don't need to feel tremendously loving to begin sex, it isn't smart to start sex when you feel disconnected or cranky toward your partner—no matter *how* horny you are. In such a situation, two people must do something to bridge the gap between feeling separated and feeling connected. If they don't, the sex will at best feel disconnected. At worst, the bodies won't cooperate and the whole thing will just feel creepy.

But even under warm and loving circumstances, people need to make the transition from not-sex to sex. Some couples have rituals, like bathing together or nibbling their favorite treats. Other couples sit together a bit and calm themselves down from the day's running around. This transition is certainly no waste of time; for many people, it's the best predictor of whether or not they will enjoy the sex that follows.

"Foreplay" is what many people call the stuff they do to make the transition from not-sex to sex (whether the sex involves intercourse or not). It may involve kissing, fondling, maybe genital play. If you don't want to do those erotic things on a given occasion, consider two more options: either do other sensual stuff that appeals to you (such as washing his hair, or licking her toes) or maybe don't have sex right now.

For many people, the longer it's been since they've had sex, the more awkward they feel when they start. That makes the transition—words, gestures, touch—even more important.

Clean up the initiation process.

In the early months of many sexual relationships, no one "initiates" sex—it "just happens" as couples make love whenever circumstances allow. After a few years that gradually stops; then someone actually has to begin the little dance each time that will culminate in either (a) two people having sex or (b) one declining the invitation.

Many people complicate this process by assigning way too much meaning to the ballet. Some people react to an invitation by thinking, "You don't realize how hard I work and how tired I get." Others believe that if a partner doesn't initiate at times when they could, it means their partner is feeling "I don't love you" or "I don't find you attractive." Some people feel they can't just say no, so they respond to an invitation with an excuse. And some people use their partner's invitation to rekindle an unfinished quarrel: "After what you said yesterday to my mother, you expect me to have sex now? Forget it."

My patients have interesting ideas about initiating sex:

- "I never initiate. When I want him to initiate, I just put on my special nightgown, and he knows tonight I'll say yes. So he initiates 100 percent of the time."

- "I know he feels pressured when I suggest sex, so I usually don't. But when we go to bed, if he lets me spoon him and doesn't move away, I figure there's a chance he might say yes."

- "I hate it when he says, 'How about tonight?' The way to let me know you're interested in sex is to shower and shave before you come to bed."

- "I'm afraid to kiss her good-night, because she'll think I'm suggesting sex. Then she complains that I never kiss her."

The rockiest part for some couples is when one partner suggests

The rockiest part for some couples is when one partner suggests sex and the other wants to decline. Every couple has to have a way for one of them to say "no thank you" without the other having bad feelings beyond mild disappointment. For too many couples "no" is usually followed by either an argument or one or more cold shoulders.

So what do you do after he or she says no to sex?

I tell some patients that the sequence of events they take for granted amazes me: "Let me get this straight. You wanted to make love with him. You wanted to create closeness and pleasure for both of you. You wanted twenty minutes that would feel special. And when he said 'no thank you,' you turned away and refused to hug, talk, or even look at him."

"That's just natural," I often hear. *No, it is not.* It's a decision that you make. A decision that does *not* enhance your relationship or your chances of creating enjoyable sex next time. And it certainly doesn't make you feel good.

Many patients struggle with what they perceive as rejection. "How would you like to be rejected? Nobody does," they wail.

"She's not rejecting you, she's rejecting sex with you," I've told many, many patients. When pressed, I say, "She didn't tell you to go away, didn't say you were disgusting, didn't say she'll never want sex with you. She just said no to sex with you in a particular moment." Of course, I encourage people who say "no thank you" to reach out and hug or touch their partner—as I remind the eager partner that this is *not* an invitation to sex.

Just as the question "do you want to go out tonight?" has many answers besides "yes" and "no" ("Yes if we can be home early," "No if you want to drink," "Only if I get a nap this afternoon," "Please ask me again after I come home from the gym"), the question "Would you like to have sex?" has many answers besides "yes" and "no." For example:

- "I'm a little tired, so I'm up for sex if you'll do most of the work."

- "Sure, if you don't mind me not climaxing."

- "Y'know, if we wait till tomorrow, I'll have a lot more energy."

- "I still have that sore on my lip, so if you can enjoy sex without kissing, okay."

- "It's already late, so could we just do a quickie?"

- "I could, but that work deadline is so much on my mind I wouldn't be there 100 percent. Do you still want to?"

Finally, making sex dates is mandatory if you have kids or other adults living in your house. Making such a date doesn't commit you to sex—after all, when the time comes you might have a headache or be cranky from taking care of a sick dog all day. Instead, you make a date to be *available* for sex. You both agree to clear your calendars for a particular time; then, if you're both in the mood, you can have sex. This avoids the complaint I hear so often, "Don't blame our lack of sex on me—I was ready last Tuesday, but you were doing email all night."

And yes, some people find the idea of planning sex so repulsive that they'd rather not have sex—and then complain about it.

Predictably, some people apparently think there's only one right way to initiate, and a partner who doesn't use it is either being disrespectful or was raised by wolves.

"Initiating" simply starts the machinery that makes the transition between sex and not-sex. Couples need to settle what that's going to look like so that they're not still arguing year after year about who should do it, or what's unromantic, or when's the best time to ask—instead of actually having sex. In fact, when couples can't work this out over time, I assume there are other unspoken things going on. I've never heard of a couple who can't eventually agree on how to discuss where to go for dinner, have you?

Take time, make time.

When you calculate the time it takes to fly across the country to visit your Aunt Minnie in her mansion (or at Graceland, in prison, at the trailer park, the Daytona Speedway—I don't know her latest gig), you know you have to include getting to the airport, hanging around after being strip-searched, and getting from the airport to your actual destination.

Similarly, the time required for sex includes time to clear your mind (of both real-world clutter and relationship clutter) and prepare your body (going to the bathroom, brushing your teeth, taking out your contact lenses). You know how it feels to be late going to the airport. Don't drag those awful emotions into your sexual experience.

Don't shortchange sex—take the time that's necessary to do it right. If you want sex but you don't have the time, enjoy a minute of kissing or fondling. Have sex later, tomorrow, or who knows when.

Focus your focus.

It's hard to *not* focus on something: Don't think of a carrot. Don't think of a carrot. Don't think of a carrot.

It's much easier to focus *on* something: think of an eggplant, all purple and shiny, with the curved stem at the top that has those grooves, and the bottom has that flattened-out leaf the same color as the stem, and if you slice it open it's not exactly white, it's more like beige, and you can see those tiny little brownish seeds.

Don't *not think* of a carrot, *think* of an eggplant.

When it comes to sex, don't tell yourself, "Don't feel nervous," or, "Don't think about success (or failure)," or, "Don't think of porn actresses." Choose your focus: your partner's body or face or skin; how you feel about him or her; how your partner's hand, mouth, hair, breasts, or weight feels on you.

Similarly, you can focus on your big belly, or on your clitoris. You can focus on your belief that your penis is too small, or you can kiss your partner and stroke her hair. You can think about the last time you had sex and felt disappointed, or you can look at your partner and say, "I'm glad we're doing this." You can—and should—focus on whatever you want during sex. Unless you're dealing with the insistent, intrusive thoughts that result from trauma, you can focus on whatever gives you enjoyment during sex.

A lot of people don't. Instead, they focus on things they find unpleasant—like self-criticism of their bodies—and then find it hard to relax during sex. That's like thinking about all the awful things they put in hot dogs while eating a hot dog, finding it hard to enjoy eating the hot dog, and then being surprised—or blaming the hot dog.

We can spoil *any* experience, whether hiking, eating, watching a movie, or playing with our kids. If you often feel, "How can I enjoy sex when I know that I'm overweight? (or wrinkled, or whatever)," you need to use some Sexual Intelligence. We don't enjoy sex because we're perfect (or because the moment is perfect or our partner is perfect), but rather despite the many imperfections built into every single sexual situation. Sexual enjoyment is not for the perfect—it's for everyone.

Don't think of a carrot, and don't *not* think of a carrot. Think of an eggplant. Or a tomato. Or any other kind of sexual experience you want to have.

Express train or local train?

Sex isn't an express train—you don't get on and then have to go to the end without stopping. That would make anyone think twice before getting (it) on.

No, sex is a local. You start, and you see how you feel. If you like it, you continue; if you don't, you change it or you stop. You get tired, you rest (you tell your partner, of course). You need to go to the bathroom, you go (you definitely tell your partner). You get a cramp, or your wrist hurts, or your jaw starts to ache, you change what you're doing. Things dry out, you get more lube or a drink of water (depending on which end is drying out).

Beginning a sexual encounter isn't a commitment to continue or "finish" it. It's a commitment to be friendly, to be open to what happens, and to communicate. This perspective may help you begin sex more frequently. Of course, it also requires that you and your partner be able to talk to each other about your experience in the moment.

Talk during sex.

Keep each other abreast of your experiences. If you're unsure where your partner is emotionally at any given time, ask. How? "Honey (huff, puff), how ya doin'?" And remember, eye contact is the ultimate "talking" during sex.

If you and your partner have talked about sex during the previous week or two, you'll have something to discuss during sex. For example, if you mentioned you were interested in the Pirate Game, or that you didn't want to try a blindfold again, you could reference that during (or after) sex.

As we discussed in Chapter 8, remember to talk about sex *outside* of bed, too.

Surprise does not equal disappointment. Disappointment does not equal failure.

On the one hand, it's fun to plan the sexual adventure you're about to have: how you're going to touch your partner, how you want to be kissed, how enthusiastic your partner will be, what a huge orgasm you're going to have, and so on. It's even more fun to talk about it with your partner ahead of time ("Tonight I'm going to caress you soooooo slowly . . . ," "On Saturday I'm going to lick you until you come big-time . . .").

That said, it's important that we not get too attached to a specific version of sex on a particular occasion, because it might not happen exactly that way.

As an analogy, imagine you're really in the mood for kung pao chicken. You say, "Let's go out for Chinese tonight; in fact, let's drive a little farther than usual and go to that place with the fabulous kung pao chicken." Your partner agrees. You drive out past the trailer park, the sagebrush, and the Liberace museum, and you arrive at Luigi's Chinese Restaurant.

You sit down, your mouth all ready for kung pao chicken, and what does the waitress with the slightly stained apron say? "By the way, no kung pao tonight. Chilis all gone." You're disappointed, of course. Your mouth was totally set for kung pao chicken. Now you have to make a decision—to enjoy the evening, ruin the evening, or go for something in between.

Notice that it's your decision, not the restaurant's.

You can leave, sulk, and go home. You can go somewhere else, but it's already getting late and the closest place is a half-hour away—besides, nobody does kung pao like Luigi. So you can stay and order any old non-kung pao thing, pick at it, and be resentful.

Or you can have a great meal. Was it the spicy heat you were looking for? You can order something with black pepper. Was it the chicken you wanted? There are lots of chicken dishes on the menu. Was it the peanuts? Get whatever you want, and ask them to add peanuts (note: not recommended in wonton soup). If you like, look at your partner and ask for a moment of sympathy over your long-lost kung pao fantasy. Then eat up, before it gets cold.

Think of sex like that—you can go in with preferences, but you must be flexible because you can't know exactly how an event is going to unfold. One of you will or won't get an erection; one of you will or won't be in the mood to play the Star Trek game; one of you will or won't want to spend as much time or energy on sex as the other; one of you will or won't get a cramp in the foot; and your partner will or won't bite you exactly where, when, and how much you want.

Fortunately, there are more ways to enjoy sex than the exact one you fantasized about. And fortunately, there's also next time.

Put orgasm in its place.

Perhaps you've noticed that I've said almost nothing about orgasm. That's because when sex is satisfying and uncomplicated, orgasm is just a small part of it. It's only when orgasm is problematic—you can't have one, or it hurts when you do, or you feel self-conscious or guilty about yours—that orgasm becomes a big part of sex.

Sex offers us a lot, including the chance to be close to someone; to give him or her gifts; to feel graceful, desired, and attractive; to discover and express ourselves; to feel special and known; to enjoy our bodies; to play games with power; and to violate taboos without penalty.

Thinking of that potential lineup puts orgasm in perspective—it's simply a bonus, and quite a brief one at that.

And although orgasm can be a wonderful, liberating moment of melting into the sun, moon, and stars (or Narnia, Hogwarts, and Middle Earth, if you prefer), it can also be bittersweet. Many people have orgasms but hardly feel them, because they're so concerned about other things, such as how long it took. For others, an orgasm is a symbol of adequacy (their own, their partner's, or both), so orgasm is something they *have*, not something they *feel*. And when sex doesn't involve much emotional connection, orgasm can be a lonely experience.

If you think orgasm is the best part of sex, you're missing a lot. And if orgasm is the only part of sex you enjoy, I imagine the rest of sex must be pretty disappointing.

So how can we make it impossible to fail at sex? By making sex more adultlike: Be sober, create a better environment, make sure you get your basic conditions met, accept yourself so your self-esteem isn't on the line, and enjoy what you get. Be disappointed—and only disappointed—when appropriate.

Or as Ashleigh Brilliant says:

"To be sure of hitting the target, shoot first, and then call whatever you hit the target."

Appendix 1

For Couples Therapists, Psychologists, and Physicians

Because Lirio's primary care physician had recently retired, his annual checkup was with someone new, a doctor who had come highly recommended. During the exam, the doctor noticed some bruises on Lirio's thighs and buttocks. Curious, he asked about them. "Oh, my boyfriend and I like to play rough," Lirio smiled. The doctor "hm-mm'd" and continued the exam. When he did Lirio's prostate exam (a lubricated, gloved finger in the rectum for two seconds), the doctor noticed some soreness, and Lirio grimaced slightly. "Take it easy there," he said. "We played just last night."

Lirio was an unusual patient: he actually talked about sex with his doctor. He didn't feel embarrassed; in fact, he felt a little bad for the doc, who was clearly uncomfortable. Lirio was used to this, though, as he taught classes in S/M and was used to encountering various attitudes about it.

The doctor was concerned, though. "Just how roughly does your partner treat you?" he asked.

Lirio explained the completely consensual domination/submission relationship he had in bed with his boyfriend Juan. It included some spanking, whipping, and anal penetration. In all of these, both he and his partner pretended Lirio was powerless, forced to "submit." I say "pretended" because Lirio and his partner had worked out the details of their game over time in a long series of conversations. Juan knew exactly what Lirio liked, what his limits were, and how to assess the impact of their play. Lirio was neither hesitant to ask for what he liked nor reluctant to say if he was too close to his limit.

So far, so good.

Except that the doc told Lirio that he looked like a victim of domestic abuse. "So I have to report this," said the doctor.

Lirio thought he must be kidding, but he wasn't. Trying to dissuade the doc, Lirio offered to call his boyfriend Juan to corroborate, but the doc wasn't interested.

Lirio then described the theory and practice of S/M. With two other patients waiting, the doctor was getting impatient. "I can't risk my family's well-being by putting my license in jeopardy," the doc said. It was surreal; Lirio was terrified. And he had only a minute or two to influence the well-meaning but naive doctor.

Suddenly Lirio had an idea. One of the office nurses seemed a little offbeat: black nail polish, a spiky leather wristband, tattoos, multiple earrings in each ear. Quickly finding her, he asked her to talk with the doctor on his behalf. It was humiliating—appealing to this stranger, who might be offended by his desperate assumption, to intervene with his own doctor, feeling like a criminal who had to marshal evidence to prevent a disaster.

The nurse turned out to be sympathetic (and into some vague S/M thing herself), and she immediately understood the importance of what Lirio was saying. She spoke with the doctor, who grudgingly dropped the whole thing. Attempting to be professional, he told Lirio, "Perhaps I'm not the right doctor for you." "We agree on that," said the relieved, stunned patient.

* * *

Lirio's story isn't unusual. In fact, data indicate that most patients involved in alternative sexual lifestyles don't trust their physician with information that's necessary for good health care. Lirio's case shows why. But let's back up a bit, and return to patients like Lirio later. First let's talk about you and me.

Most clinicians get little or no training in sexuality (for example, California social workers are only required to take a single, ten-hour seminar). The training we do get is typically pathology-oriented: sex abuse, "sex addiction," sexual violence, HIV rates, unintended pregnancy, sex tourism and trafficking. There's rarely a mention of pleasure, the clitoris, or healthy non-monogamy.

And there's rarely a mention of the enormous range of human sexual behaviors, unless it's in the context of pathology ("a wide array of fetishes and paraphilias are known"). You can get licensed as a physician, marriage counselor, nurse, or social worker without ever hearing about, much less seeing, a vibrator.

This is bad for us both professionally and personally. It's bad for our patients, too.

But it does mirror how most of our patients learn about sexuality: the theme is generally danger and fear, with rumors of orgiastic pleasure thrown in (without, of course, much instruction for bringing that about).

We've already seen that the Sexual Intelligence approach is the opposite of what most patients learn and experience. In many ways, it's also the opposite of what professionals learn in our training. This appendix examines (and critiques) common responses to patients with sexual issues, and describes how a Sexual Intelligence approach can serve them better.

And if we grow ourselves while treating patients in a more sophisticated, humane way, that's okay too. Everyone benefits when a professional gains a little Sexual Intelligence.

Noticing Our Assumptions so We Can Minimize Them

Most psychologists and physicians live in the same culture as their patients—they watch the same TV shows, use the same smartphone apps, even go to the same church or gym.

A lot of our patients' sexual (and relationship) difficulties are a direct result of their assumptions—about men, women, sex, love, intimacy, desire, and bodies. Patients typically hold certain problematic beliefs: that women should climax from intercourse; that erections should be ready-on-demand regardless of how a man feels; that desire is a natural outgrowth of love; that heterosexuals don't (and shouldn't) enjoy same-sex fantasies; and that sex should be natural and spontaneous. Beliefs like these undergird many common sexual difficulties.

Thus, *a major part of successful treatment involves helping patients see their assumptions,* discussing their unwanted consequences, and exploring alternative beliefs.

However, if we ourselves can't see our patients' assumptions, we obviously can't point them out. And to the extent that we share those assumptions, it will be almost impossible to see them in a patient. Do you ever notice how everyone around you believes in gravity? No? Ever notice that people believe rain is wet? No? Ever notice that other people don't eat soup with a knife? No? When we live as others do, it's hard to notice what they do. Fish, as they say, don't realize they live in water.

So if we as therapists and health care providers think that sex equals intercourse, we won't notice when patients think so. If we think it's unsexy or unromantic to use lubricants and condoms, or make dates for sex, we won't notice when patients do. If we think that telling a partner what you like in bed is being bossy, we won't notice when patients have the same attitude. What we don't notice will make it impossible for us to diagnose, or to challenge such beliefs as the source of problems.

Thus, it's crucial for us to know what our *own* sexual assumptions are. We don't necessarily have to change them, but we need to know what they are, and we need to know that they're not "right," but merely a single point of view.

This presents a challenge not just to clinicians' professional values but to their *personal* values and assumptions as well.

How Our Values Shape Our Work

As competent adult members of American culture, every therapist and physician has ideas about various aspects of sexuality. Is it okay for married people to masturbate? How much masturbation is "excessive"? Is homosexuality "normal"? How much sexual desire is "reasonable"? Is getting turned on by spanking "too kinky"? Like sexual variety itself, the questions are endless.

Note that there are no "right" or "scientific" answers to these questions. They refer to issues of values, not of fact. All of us have a sense of what's "normal," "right," and "real" about sex, even if we don't realize it. This sense about sexuality is such a deep part of our reality that it can be invisible to us—even when we're conveying that sense as part of our clinical work.

Consider a few simple examples: We generally assume that married patients are monogamous. We often assume that a woman who's had an abortion feels guilty or grief-stricken. We may ask patients their age when they first "had sex"—without specifying whether we mean partner sex, and if so, whether we mean intercourse (many people have oral sex or anal sex for years before first intercourse). And we may forget to ask if the sex was consensual, coercive, or something in between—a big lapse considering that a substantial number of first sexual experiences are not fully consensual.

Here are examples of values issues that shape our work—the questions we ask, our interpretations of the answers, and our suggestions based on those interpretations:

- What is "normal" sexuality?

- Sexually, what are "men" and "women" like?

- What is "normal" desire? What drives it?

- What is the relationship of fantasy, desire, and arousal?

- Can kinky sex be healthy? Can it involve intimacy?

- Can desires to surrender or dominate be healthy?

- What is the relationship between sex, love, and intimacy?

- What is the meaning of adult masturbation? What is its role in a relationship?

Note that it is primarily our *non-professional* ideas about these issues that shape our *professional* thinking and behavior: partly because we don't get specialized training in sexuality, but also because we develop ideas about sexuality as ordinary adults in society. We wouldn't make a similar professional leap in other areas in which we have no expertise—say, roofing or auto repair—even if we had opinions or general ideas as laypeople. Unfortunately, the clinical professions undervalue real expertise in sexuality; "reasonable" lay opinions in fancy language are more or less the state of the art.

And so we intervene in cases based on our ideas about, say, sexual submission (politically incorrect for women), exhibitionism (juvenile, hostile), casual sex (fear of intimacy), pornography (degrading to women, even when it shows women having pleasure), affairs ("sex addiction"), or same-gender fantasies ("latent homosexuality"). While each of these interpretations will be accurate for some patients, they will be wildly inaccurate for many others. If you walk into the consulting room with preconceived ideas like these, you'll be ignoring the reality of a substantial number of your patients. Your world may feel validated, but theirs won't. At least a quarter of my new patients are refugees from this sort of demeaning professional treatment.

Again, it doesn't matter so much what your answers to values questions are; what matters is your awareness that you have those answers, that they're probably based on your non-professional life, and that they shape your professional behavior without you realizing it. That's what should grab your attention. And then every professional should spend some time identifying just what their sexual values are.

Sexual Function vs. Sexual Enjoyment

Some patients are very tangible in describing what they want from sex. They want better erections, or quicker lubrication, they want to last longer or climax quicker, they want more desire. Or they want their partner to change in these ways. They want someone's "dysfunction" fixed, either their own or their partner's.

If we choose, a good therapist or physician can investigate a patient's life and often uncover the logic (conscious or unconscious) that makes sense of these "symptoms": trauma, fear of abandonment, insecurity about masculinity, fear of intimacy—the whole Oprah-ocracy of inner torment we regularly see.

Given America's twisted sexual culture, if we're looking for stuff like that, we can almost always find it. Then, theoretically, we help our patients resolve it, the blocks to sexual function dissolve, and their genitalia are rescued from the ash heap of history. Good-bye, sexual "dysfunction."

Whether that's the best we can do for our patients is another matter.

I'm not so eager to agree that I'll work with a patient to fix presenting problems like unreliable erections and discouraged vaginas. When I ask patients why these symptoms are a problem, their answers are often interesting, such as:

- "I'm afraid my partner will leave me."

- "I don't feel like a real man."

- "It means God is angry that I masturbate."

- "I'm afraid I'm gay."

- "It means there's something wrong with me."

- "I'm afraid it means I don't love my partner."

- "I don't want to get old."

- "I'm afraid my partner will punish me."

- "How will I ever find a partner, given my emotional baggage?"

I tell new patients that these aren't sex problems. They're insecurity, existential challenges, relationship problems, and misunderstandings about the nature of intimacy. Problems like these won't be fixed by curing their sexual symptoms. Just as importantly, fixing their genitalia isn't the key to the great sex that people say they want.

Professionals need to help people have better *enjoyment* rather than better *functioning.*

I approach sexual "function" as a means, not an end in itself. So memo to clinicians: quit working so hard to fix people's erection, lubrication, and orgasm problems! Start dealing with their real difficulties: their perfectionism and resulting alienation from their bodies, their unrealistic expectations, their small-minded vision of sexuality, their performance anxiety.

It's true, of course, that there are physiological problems that create sexual symptoms.

Some patients absolutely need a medical workup: those with shortness of breath (co-occurs with erection problems) and heavy menstrual bleeding (co-occurs with painful intercourse), to name just two. We want to make sure every patient has had a basic blood workup done within our lifetime; hypothyroidism and low testosterone or estrogen levels can create a wide range of mischief. When new middle-aged patients say that they haven't seen a doctor in six years, I tell them they'll need to do that as part of our treatment.

But diagnostically, let's start simple. Remember: when you hear hooves, think horses, not zebras.

I've had dozens of new patients report that they received a prescription for an erection drug without being asked how they felt about their partner (many of them found their wives or girlfriends unappealing). I've known doctors to treat chronic yeast infections without finding out that, although the patient was having sex with her husband only every few months, she was regularly sleeping with someone else.

Finding out about our patients' lives is a key part of treating their sexual issues. Or rather, it's a key part of discovering which sexual issues need treating.

Identify Patients' Sexual Narratives

As we've already seen, narratives are the stories that patients tell themselves (some consciously, others unconsciously) about who they are, what they can expect from sex, and what various experiences mean.

Some people have positive or neutral sexual narratives: I am attractive, capable, desirable. Or I'm good enough, I'm regular, I'm more or less normal. But people like this usually don't come to our offices with sexual distress.

Instead, we see patients who think of themselves as damaged, inadequate, unattractive, godforsaken, old, blameworthy—in short, unsexy and ineligible for being desired or sexually satisfied.

This narrative itself can be critical to helping patients change their sexual experience. Addressing this narrative, rather than the balky vagina or penis or the elusive climax, is often the key.

Of course, it isn't enough to say, "You think you're damaged, but you're not!" or, "You may feel unattractive, but I think you're attractive!" You might as well tell a depressed person, "Have a nice day!" and expect it to lift their depression.

No, our job is more subtle. First we have to explain to patients what a narrative is; then we have to describe (to mirror) what their narrative is; then we have to help them investigate how their narrative undermines their sexual satisfaction; then we have to help them see that their narrative is a choice; and finally we have to help them weave a different narrative—one of adequacy and eligibility, one based on Sexual Intelligence rather than on killer abs or perfect breasts.

Deferring Too Much to Culture

America is far more conscious of its diversity now than ever before. So after decades of unconsciously imagining the "average" patient (white, middle-class, monogamous, sober), clinicians are now far more sensitive to the idiosyncratic cultural issues that accompany each new patient. "Diversity" is this decade's big theme in both clinical and corporate training—what "don't be a sexist pig" was three decades ago.

Nevertheless, while being sensitive to people's individuality and idiosyncratic biographies, we don't want to ignore our best tools or to make assumptions about our patients' limitations. It's true that, say, Asian people *tend* to be more private about their sexuality than Caucasians. And fundamentalist Christians *tend* to assume that women will submit to their husband's sexual desires. And orthodox Jews *generally* believe masturbation is a sin. And, and, and. . . .

But we also don't want to stereotype people and cultures like we did in third grade. (You remember: "Holland: wooden shoes. India: elephants and tigers. Russia: drunk, impotent men.") We want to walk a fine line: to be culturally sensitive without withholding our best work because we prejudge that people won't be able to hear or value what we say.

This is especially true regarding religion. Inflexibility is inflexibility, regardless of the source. We can be respectful of patients' beliefs *and* discuss the inevitable consequences of them at the same time. If, for example, a man believes it's a sin to fantasize about women he sees on the street, that's his right—but it's going to make sex very complicated for him, and he deserves our best clinical insight about that. Similarly, if people insist that the only acceptable birth control is withdrawal before ejaculation, or that there are only a few days per month when a woman is clean enough to have intercourse, that's their right—but that makes sex very complicated for them. We owe our patients clear information.

Here in Silicon Valley, I work with a lot of people who were born in Asia, or whose parents were born there. As a result, I periodically see patients involved with arranged marriages. Half of these people know their prospective spouse for months or even years; the other half meet their mate only weeks or even hours before the wedding.

Baldev and Gita both grew up in the coastal area of southern India. Their families had betrothed them in their early teens, and they married as college freshmen—having spent virtually no time together unchaperoned. Now in their mid-twenties, they'd been having sexual difficulties from the very start of their marriage. In addition, she wasn't pregnant yet, and their families were pressuring them. "Don't be a typical American," his mother warned her, "postponing childbearing until you can only have one or two."

As a Westerner, I find arranged marriage to be an alien institution, of course. But my patients and a half-dozen teaching trips across Asia have taught me a lot about its advantages and disadvantages. If Baldev and Gita had still been in India, they might have consulted with older siblings, clan elders, maybe a priest or doctor of traditional Ayurvedic medicine.

Here in California, they chose to see me. So how do we work with such people struggling with sexual difficulties?

After detailing their marital history, I looked at them and said, "You know, I'm not Indian." They smiled at my small joke and relaxed a bit. "So I'm no expert on arranged marriages. But I do know a little bit, and you'll tell me the rest of what I need to know.

"I appreciate that both your families were involved in your relationship even before it started," I said. "So in a sense there are more than two of you in this marriage." They nodded. "When we talk about sex, we usually think of the two people who are actually making love. But in your case that would be simplistic. Both your families were involved in the betrothal, the courtship, the wedding—two, three days, I bet, what an event!—and the honeymoon. Eagerly awaiting your first child, they've been in your bedroom ever since. This isn't a criticism," I emphasized, "just a description. Please tell me what this has been like for you."

They were polite, a bit shy, and spoke in generalities and euphemisms. So I supplied a few words to help the conversation along. "I think almost any man would have trouble getting an erection if he felt people were looking over his shoulder," I suggested. I gently continued, "And most women would find it hard to relax and let go if they imagined their mother or father in the next room." I let my words sink in.

"Yes," Baldev said quietly, "that's kind of how it was. I think maybe you felt that way too, Gita?" Of course she did. So I went a step further.

"You're both engineers, right? You know, it's one thing to set people loose in a lab and tell them to work on a project. But imagine if they don't know how to use the equipment, have no experience, don't know each other well, are on a deadline—and they're expected to work in the dark! How would that be?" They looked a little confused, so I spelled it out for them.

"You two were sent into a lab—your marital bed. Neither of you had any experience, you knew nothing about each other's body, you didn't know each other well enough to work as a team, and you felt you had to create a result—successful sex—on schedule. And to make it even harder to learn anything, you believed you had to do it in the dark!"

Their dark eyes opened wide as the accuracy of the description touched them. "And," I concluded softly, "you've been operating under this kind of pressure, week after week, ever since. It must be a terrible strain."

Gita was the first to speak. "I feel I've disappointed you many times," she said to Baldev. "No, no," her husband responded. "I've not been the man who . . . who . . . ," he choked back tears. "It's all my fault."

And that was the beginning of a series of very productive, if painful, sessions. Years of frustration, shame, and self-criticism— all suffered in emotional isolation from each other—suddenly had a voice. It was as if they were each discovering that they had a partner for the first time.

The expectations each had felt were such a burden.

> "I thought I was supposed to excite you, but I didn't know how—and I know my breasts are very small."

> "I heard there was something down there I was supposed to touch, but I couldn't find it!"

> "I hear other women love to . . . you know, orally satisfy the husband. . . . I didn't know how to start, and I was afraid to hurt you."

> "I felt you were depending on me, and I wanted to succeed so much, and I felt so embarrassed."

They were still young, and they did care for each other, and they were bright and open. And so a little information, a lot of communication, and the encouragement to begin their sexual relationship all over—starting with holding hands, kissing, and a couple of lingering pats on the behind—went a long way. After a few months, they waved good-bye to me, erotically more confident (in a sweetly shy way) and feeling more in charge of their lives than they'd ever imagined.

And although these details might be dramatically different than in the case of an American couple raised with sex, drugs, and rock 'n' roll, the issues with most of my patients are similar: harsh expectations, inadequate information, emotional isolation, performance pressure, intercourse orientation, and the trivialization of individual sexual scripts.

By the way, when I teach in Asia I talk about changing the meaning of the Wedding Night: from "first intercourse" to "launching the couple's sexual career, with touching and talking." It's a hard sell in traditional, procreation-oriented cultures, but I'm trying.

"Alternative" Sexuality

Whether we know it or not, a lot of our patients express their sexuality outside of traditional boundaries. They're into S/M, threesomes, commercial sex, chat rooms, semi-public sex, swing clubs, and fetishes like gloves (rubber, leather, lace) or high heels (their own or others'; kissing them, wearing them, being stepped on by them). And of course our patients are involved with taboo activities that are hardly non-traditional—affairs and pornography, for example.

So how do we deal with these forms of sexual expressions? Without special training, we rely on what we already have—our own beliefs (prejudices?), our own experiences (positive or negative), and the vaguely suspicious, slightly negative, and altogether conventional sexual attitude of our profession.

Psychologists are committed to looking beyond the content of patients' stories and lives, and focusing on situational and psychological dynamics. But this commitment often dwindles when the subject is sex. Whereas we don't usually tell patients how to run their lives, we often tell them what not to do sexually; whereas we don't usually tell them whether one or another approach to life is "normal" (even if they ask!), we eagerly opine on the normality of their sex lives—frequently pathologizing what they do or desire.

Physicians have learned to talk to patients about lifestyle trade-offs; for example, orthopedists routinely tell patients that if tennis brings them pleasure, maybe accepting a little knee pain is a good choice. While doctors generally look to patients' values and lifestyle when considering interventions, they are often too uncomfortable to do that regarding sex, substituting moralizing for medicine.

Many patients live with years of secrecy and shame, which almost always hurts them far more than whatever their sexual preferences are. I see men tearfully confess to masturbating into their wife's panties, for example, and women anxiously confess to thinking about another woman in order to climax with a boyfriend. Decades of hiding and feeling guilty undermine both sexual function and intimacy. Often, such people lose their desire because, unconsciously, it's the easiest way to distance themselves from their pain.

When patients ask us to fix their sexuality, we should go very, very slowly. Our initial goal should be sympathizing with their secrecy and shame, not changing their sexual expression. If the latter comes up at all—and it may not, if we effectively treat their emotional pain—it should be at the end of treatment, not the beginning.

We also need to understand that many aspects of "alternative" relationships are not necessarily about the sexual dynamic. When couples who happily swing can't agree on whether their kid should have to earn his allowance or get it free, or on how to deal with the in-laws, or what to do about one of them being chronically late, their swinging is probably irrelevant. People into sexual expressions like bisexuality, S/M, or role-playing have the same rest-of-a-life that more traditional people have. So when faced with a patient involved in alternative sexual experiences, don't be too quick to make that the centerpiece of the patient's life or your treatment. However difficult it is, don't let your own discomfort undermine the helpful neutrality that all patients need.

When This Approach
Challenges the Clinician

Since most clinicians are marinating in the same distorted, sex-negative culture as our patients, we should assume that we've all internalized some version of the limited belief system about "normal sex" and "performance" that haunts our patients. And so, if we successfully challenge our patients' allegiance to this way of thinking, we will inevitably confront our own allegiance to the same dysfunctional ideas.

This can be quite spectacular.

You might actually become aware of your own "ineligible/inadequate" narrative. You might realize that you feel resentful or self-critical about the ways in which you've accepted others' limitations of your sexuality, or imposed limitations on yourself. You might discover that you're still in some sexual closet or other regarding your mate.

You might become jealous of patients who liberate themselves. You might resent their spouses who try to prevent that. You might become nervous about the impulses inside you that you've safely tucked away as impractical, not normal, or not real. And you might feel grief—over what you've given up, sold too cheaply, or done without realizing it.

Grief is an important stage in eventually appreciating who we have become, and what's now available for us to pursue. Everyone's afraid to grieve, although we all want the serenity and energy on the other side of grief. You know, "Everyone wants to get to heaven, but nobody wants to die. . . ."

Appendix 2

Hand Massage: An Exercise

Decide who will be partner A and who will be partner B. It doesn't matter which is which.

This assignment takes five minutes. Please do it without the radio or TV on, when you have a bit of privacy, and away from your cell phones. Use some hand lotion—any brand or type is fine. Start by washing and drying your hands. Then each person should rub a tiny bit of lotion on their own hands, just to smooth out any rough spots.

A, take one of B's hands in yours. Rub that hand *for your own pleasure and interest*. Perhaps you want to check out the fingernails or calluses or plump places. You may want to rub the hand vigorously or gently, or alternate. B, *don't say or indicate anything*—no sighs or faces or words of encouragement—unless it hurts or tickles. In that case, please say so, and if so, A should change what she/he is doing.

A, rub this hand for one minute. Look at it while you're doing so. After a minute, put this hand down, and take B's other hand. Rub this hand for a minute, but this time do it *for B's pleasure and enjoyment*. B, this time *use words or sounds* to let A know how you like what she or he is doing. Don't tell A what to do, just respond to what A is doing so that A knows whether to continue or to change. A, respond to B's feedback, while also rubbing this hand in the various ways that occur to you. After one minute, put this hand down.

Then switch—B, take one of A's hands and rub it according to your own interests. After a minute, take A's other hand and rub it with the goal of giving him or her enjoyment. Remember to look at the hand you're rubbing.

Afterwards, say a few words to each other about some aspect of your experience. If you both want to have a longer conversation, go ahead. At the very least, each of you should say one thing that was interesting about this time together.

Marty Klein, Ph.D.

Certified Sex Therapist
Licensed Marriage and Family Therapist

2439 Birch Street, #2
Palo Alto, CA 94306
650-856-6533
Klein@SexEd.org